Edited by

WILLIAM L. MEYERHOFF, M.D., Ph.D.

Professor and Chairman
Department of Otolaryngology
University of Texas Health Science Center at Dallas
Southwestern Medical School

Assistant Editors:

STEPHEN LISTON, M.D.

Assistant Professor
Department of Otolaryngology
University of Minnesota Medical School

ROBERT G. ANDERSON, M.D.

Assistant Professor
Department of Otorhinolaryngology
University of Texas Health Science Center at Dallas
Southwestern Medical School

DIAGNOSIS AND MANAGEMENT OF

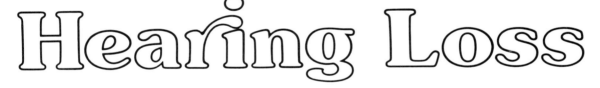

W. B. SAUNDERS COMPANY_____1984

Philadelphia   London   Toronto
Mexico City   Rio de Janeiro   Sydney   Tokyo

W. B. Saunders Company: West Washington Square
                          Philadelphia, PA 19105

                          1 St. Anne's Road
                          Eastbourne, East Sussex BN21 3UN, England

                          1 Goldthorne Avenue
                          Toronto, Ontario M8Z 5T9, Canada

                          Apartado 26370—Cedro 512
                          Mexico 4, D.F., Mexico

                          Rua Coronel Cabrita, 8
                          Sao Cristovao Caixa Postal 21176
                          Rio de Janeiro, Brazil

                          9 Waltham Street
                          Artarmon, N.S.W. 2064, Australia

                          Ichibancho, Central Bldg., 22-1 Ichibancho
                          Chiyoda-Ku, Tokyo 102, Japan

Library of Congress Cataloging in Publication Data

Meyerhoff, William L.

Diagnosis and management of hearing loss.

1. Deafness.   I. Title.   II. Title: Hearing loss. [DNLM: 1.
Hearing disorders—Diagnosis.   2. Hearing disorders—
Therapy.   WV 270 M6135d]

RF290.M49   1984   617.8   83-20416
ISBN 0–7216–1307–1

Diagnosis and Management of Hearing Loss   ISBN 0-7216-1307-1

Last digit is the print number: 9   8   7   6   5   4   3   2   1

To my father, without whose help my education would have stopped many years ago; and to my mother, wife, and three daughters for their constant support.

CONTRIBUTORS

ROBERT G. ANDERSON, M.D.
Assistant Professor, Department of Otorhinolaryngology, University of Texas
Health Science Center at Dallas, Dallas, Texas

RENÉ BOOTHBY, M.D.
Stanford University Medical Center, Division of Otolaryngology, Stanford,
California

JOSEPH B. CARTER, M.D.
Department of Otolaryngology, Euclid Clinic Foundation, Euclid, Ohio

LARRY G. DUCKERT, M.D., Ph.D.
Associate Professor, Department of Otolaryngology, University of Washington
School of Medicine, Seattle, Washington

MARCOS V. GOYCOOLEA, M.D., Ph.D.
Dirección General Estudiantil, Catholic University of Chile; Chile Military
Hospital, Santiago, Chile

EARL R. HARFORD, Ph.D.
Professor, Department of Otolaryngology, University of Minnesota Medical
School, Minneapolis, Minnesota

PETER HILGER, M.D., Ph.D.
Assistant Professor, Department of Otolaryngology, University of Minnesota
Medical School, Minneapolis, Minnesota

DAVID W. JOHNSON, M.S., M.A., C.C.C.
Clinical Audiologist, Hennepin County Medical Center, Minneapolis, Minnesota

STEPHEN LISTON, M.D.
Assistant Professor, Department of Otolaryngology, University of Minnesota
Medical School, Minneapolis, Minnesota

WILLIAM L. MEYERHOFF, M.D.
Professor and Chairman, Department of Otolaryngology, University of Texas
Health Science Center at Dallas, Dallas, Texas

MICHAEL M. PAPARELLA, M.D.
Professor and Chairman, Department of Otolaryngology, University of Minnesota Medical School, Minneapolis, Minnesota

DONALD W. SHREWSBURY, M.D.
Tacoma, Washington

HUBERT VERMEERSCH, M.D.
Akademisch Ziedenhuis, Neus-, Keel- EN Oorkliniek, Gent, Belgium

PREFACE

The objective of this text is to provide a logical and comprehensive approach to the understanding of hearing loss and related conditions. The first step toward achieving this objective is to recognize the spectrum of the problem and then to gather knowledgeable experts who can address individual aspects in a clear and concise manner. The psychosocial, educational, and economic scopes of hearing loss are put into perspective in Chapter 1, which also provides a foundation for the science of hearing as well as a system for categorizing hearing loss and an approach to patients suffering this malady. Chapter 2 discusses congenital hearing loss from etiologic and therapeutic standpoints, and Chapter 3 provides an in-depth understanding of otitis media, the most common cause of conductive hearing loss. Chapter 4 covers sensorineural hearing loss, and Chapter 5 discusses a particularly frightening form of sensorineural hearing loss, that which occurs suddenly. In Chapter 6, current knowledge of tinnitus, a most perplexing symptom, is detailed, and the incapacitating symptom of vertigo is addressed in Chapter 7. Audiologic aspects of hearing loss are covered in Chapter 8, and methods of screening and their rationale are outlined in Chapter 9.

It is the editor's hope that this text will serve to enhance the education of audiologists, medical students, family practitioners, and otolaryngologists during their residency and early years of practice in this rapidly changing field. This endeavor, of course, could in no way be achieved without the excellent help, patience, and cooperation extended by the assistant editors and contributors.

CONTENTS

William L. Meyerhoff
Joseph B. Carter

1

SCOPE OF THE PROBLEM AND FUNDAMENTALS

Hearing loss may be the most common physical disability suffered by people living in the United States. If affects between 13 and 22 million Americans, 6 million of whom are profoundly deaf. Hearing impairment gives rise to educational, economic, and psychosocial handicaps. The commonly associated otologic dysfunctions that cause tinnitus and vertigo compound the physical handicap, the psychologic impairment, and the socioeconomic impact. Successful management of the problems associated with hearing loss requires an understanding of the underlying pathophysiology. Hearing loss is a symptom, not a diagnosis, and in every case a thorough medical evaluation is mandatory in an effort to identify the underlying cause and to direct individualized treatment and rehabilitation. Understanding this basic concept is especially important when dealing with patients manifesting sensorineural hearing loss.

The Magnitude of the Problem

The true prevalence of hearing loss and its impact are difficult to assess. It is important to clarify the terminology because its misuse has contributed to inaccuracies in expressing the magnitude of the problem. *Hearing impairment* is a deviation or a change for the worse in auditory function, usually outside the range of normal. *Functional hearing impairment* is an impairment without an organic basis. A *hearing handicap* is a disadvantage imposed by an impairment that is severe enough to affect one's personal efficiency in the activities of daily living. A *hearing disability* is an impairment that results in actual or presumed inability to remain employed at full wages (Table 1–1). Using these criteria, it is estimated that approximately 8 per cent of the population of the United States suffer some hearing handicap, and approximately 3 per cent of the population suffer a severe handicap. Between 2000 and 4000 profoundly deaf children are born each year, representing about 0.1 per cent of all newborns. One per cent of adolescents, 2 per cent of adults, 30 per cent of people over the age of 65, and 50 per cent of people over 85 years of age have significant hearing handicaps.

The interrelationships between the ear and the brain are the most highly developed of any sensory system. Unfortunately our understanding of these interrelationships is not complete. Hearing is an interpretive ability as well as a receptive sense. Not all individuals respond in the same way to similar impairments, and, therefore, experts cannot really specify the total capabilities of the hearing mechanism. Similarly, in different people, the same handicap may not create the same disability. Hearing levels sufficient for one occupation might prove inadequate for another. The direct and indirect financial costs associated with hearing loss in the areas of education, employment, and social service are unknown but are substantial to both the individual and society.

The psychological effects associated with hearing impairment can be severe and include frustration, suspicion, fear, loss of pride, shame, and withdrawal from society.

1

Table 1–1. FORMULA FOR CALCULATING PERCENTAGE DISABILITY DUE TO HEARING LOSS

I. Calculate average threshold (AT) for hearing in both the best hearing ear and the worst hearing ear by adding the thresholds at 500 Hz, 1000 Hz, 2000 Hz, and 4000 Hz and dividing the sum by 4.

II. Calculate monaural impairment (MI) by subtracting 25 dB from the calculated AT in each ear and multiply the difference by 1.5 per cent. If the difference is less than zero (negative difference), the MI for that ear is considered zero. If the MI for both ears is zero, there is no hearing disability.

III. Calculate percentage hearing disability by multiplying the MI in the better hearing ear by 5, adding that product to the MI in the worst ear, and dividing the sum by 6. The quotient equals the percentage disability.

Examples

A. Unilateral HL*

	500 Hz	1000 Hz	2000 Hz	4000 Hz
AS†	5 dB	10 dB	10 dB	20 dB
AD‡	40 dB	45 dB	50 dB	75 dB

1. Calculate Average Threshold
   AS = (5 + 10 + 10 + 20)/4 = 45/4 = 11 dB
   AD = (40 + 45 + 50 + 75)/4 = 210/4 = 53 dB

2. Calculate Monaural Impairment
   AS = 11 dB − 25 dB = 14 (considered zero) × 1.5%
   AD = 53 − 25 dB = 28 dB; 28 dB × 1.5% − 42%

3. Calculate Percentage Hearing Disability
   AS (better hearing ear) = 0 × 5 = 0
   AD (poorer hearing ear) = 42 × 1 = 42%
                  Sum =   42%
   Disability 42 ÷ 6   =   7%

   The hearing disability for this patient = 7%

B. Bilateral HL

	500 Hz	1000 Hz	2000 Hz	4000 Hz
AS	35 dB	30 dB	45 dB	60 dB
AD	35 dB	35 dB	45 dB	60 dB

1. Calculate Average Threshold
   AS = (35 + 30 + 45 + 60)/4 = 105/4 = 43 dB
   AD = (35 + 35 + 45 + 60)/4 = 175/4 = 44 dB

2. Calculate Monaural Impairment
   AS = 43 dB − 25 dB = 18 dB; 18 × 1.5% = 27%
   AD = 44 dB − 25 dB = 19 dB; 19 × 1.5% = 29%

3. Calculate Percentage Hearing Disability
   AS (better hearing ear) = 27% × 5 = 135
   AD (worse hearing ear) = 29% × 1 = 29
                  Sum =   164
   Disability   = 164 ÷ 6 = 27%

   The hearing disability for this patient = 27%

*HL = Hearing loss.
†AS = Left ear.
‡AD = Right ear.

Psychological maladjustments may be particularly severe if the loss occurs rapidly or at the extremes of age. Developmental problems may be expected when the hearing loss is congenital or occurs at a young age. Hearing loss occurring in young adulthood and in middle life may shatter career plans. Hearing impairment may result in isolation and loneliness, especially in the elderly.

The hearing impaired individual is faced with a dual handicap. The hearing loss represents not only a communication handicap but also an underlying auditory pathologic condition. To effectively understand and assist the victims of hearing impairment, we must reach a better understanding of these underlying pathologic mechanisms.

Basic Terminology

Sound is the propagation of a mechanical disturbance through an elastic medium.

Sound energy generated by a physical disturbance results in an alteration of the propagating medium. Local areas of increased and decreased pressure arise and are transmitted through the medium as a sound wave. The characteristics of this energy wave are determined by the density, mass, and temperature of the medium as well as the characteristics of the disturbing mechanism.

Two dimensions that are important in the description of sound energy are *intensity* (I) and *frequency* (F). Intensity is the physical measurement of the rate of energy flow per unit area and is expressed in units of watts per cm². In audiology, *pressure* (P) is a more commonly used dimension because it is more convenient to measure than intensity. Pressure represents a quantity of force per unit area and is directly proportional to the square root of the intensity. *Loudness* is the perceived or psychoacoustic correlate of intensity and pressure. The relationship between pressure, or intensity, and loudness is not linear. The dynamic range of the hearing mechanism from the threshold of audibility to the threshold of discomfort represents about 15 orders of magnitude of intensity (or seven and one-half orders of magnitude of pressure). Because of this tremendous range, it is convenient to specify the intensity of a given sound in a logarithmic fashion and to compare it with a known standard. This logarithmic ratio is known as a bel in honor of Alexander Graham Bell. However, for practical applications, the use of the *decibel* (dB), a unit of one tenth of a bel, is more satisfactory. The term decibel is used in many different situations, but it always compares the intensity or pressure of one signal with the intensity or pressure of a second signal. Thus, by definition, one sound with intensity I1 is x decibels more intense than a sound with intensity I2 when

$$x = 10 \log \frac{I1}{I2}$$

When decibels are described in terms of pressure ratios rather than intensity ratios then

$$x = \log \frac{P1}{P2}$$

Although pressure is only proportionally equal to the square root of intensity, both formulas are equally valid because the proportionally constant, which is the reciprocal of the characteristic impedance of the propagating medium, cancels out in the ratios of the two pressures. Since decibel notation implies a ratio, it is important to specify the reference level (I2 or P2). Some reference levels are abbreviated because of their common usage. The most commonly used reference is that of an intensity of 10 watts per cm², which is equivalent to 0.0002 dynes per cm² of pressure air. When this reference level is used, the signal is expressed in terms of sound pressure level (SPL or dB SPL). Hearing level (HTL or dB HL) refers to an internationally derived reference determined by the average threshold of a population of normal-hearing subjects at a given frequency. Sensation level (dB SL) utilizes the threshold of a given subject at the signal frequency as the reference level. Other references may be used, but they must always be specified.

The other important dimension in describing an auditory signal is the frequency composition of the signal. The term frequency defines the duration of each period of vibration of the sound energy. The most elementary example is that of a sinusoidal signal or pure tone, such as that created by the simple harmonic motion of a tuning fork or by an electronic oscillator. These tones may easily be assigned a frequency by determining the number of repetitions or cycles occurring per unit of time. Frequency is expressed in units of cycles per second or hertz (Hz). Few naturally occurring sounds can be described as pure tones. Most are brief atonal sounds known as transients. All sounds, however, can be described in terms of their frequency content, as if they consisted of an algebraic sum of a number of pure tones.

Pitch is the psychological correlate of frequency. The relationship between frequency and pitch is quite complex. Signals with greatly disparate frequency compositions may evoke a similar pitch. Pitch is a subjective phenomenon and is an area of intense investigation.

Anatomy and Physiology of Hearing

The human ear is a remarkable instrument. It usually performs its task of gathering the pressure fluctuations of an acoustic signal and transforming the information into a series of neural impulses quite efficiently. The human ear can respond to frequencies between 15 and 20,000 Hz, although the high-frequency performance deteriorates with age. The ear displays a dynamic range of about 130 dB between the weakest signal threshold and the level of signal sufficient to cause pain.

PERIPHERAL AND CENTRAL SYSTEMS

When discussing the anatomy and physiology of the ear, it is convenient to divide the auditory system into peripheral and central components. The peripheral component consists of three subsystems: the outer, middle, and inner ear. The auditory nerve (cranial nerve VIII) is often, on clinical grounds, considered part of the peripheral system as well. The central system includes the brainstem cochlear nuclei, superior olive, lateral lemniscus, inferior colliculus, medial geniculate body, auditory representation in the cerebral cortex, and a diversity of interconnections and pathways. Sound awareness may be, at least in part, a brainstem phenomenon, although most of the appreciation of sound, its pitch, intensity, and discrimination, occurs in the temporal lobe of the cerebral cortex. Central auditory function and dysfunction are currently subjects of intense and exciting research.

External Ear

The most lateral component in the peripheral auditory system, the external ear, consists of the pinna or auricle, the external auditory meatus, and the external auditory canal. The auricle is composed of fibroelastic cartilage and is attached to the skull by the overlying skin, an extension of cartilage into the external auditory canal, three ligaments (anterior, posterior, and superior), and three muscles (anterior, posterior, and superior). Embryologically it is derived from six hillocks of His, which are primordial elevations on the first (mandibular) and second (hyoid) branchial arches. The auricle receives sensory innervation from cranial nerves V, VII, and X as well as from the upper two cervical rootlets. The three muscles receive their motor innervation from cranial nerve VII. As can be seen in Figure 1–1, the contour of the pinna includes complicated convolutions. The most frequent deformity is lop ear, caused by the underdevelopment of the

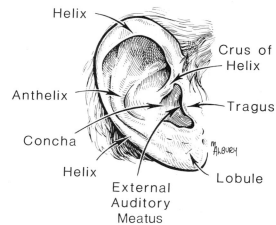

Figure 1–1. Normal human ear.

antihelical fold and prominence of the caudihelix (Fig. 1–2).

The most important functional property of the external ear is the role it plays in sound localization. Although not well developed in humans, the pinna may be extremely useful in directional hearing in animals such as the dog or the horse.

The external auditory canal ranges in length from about 2.3 to 2.9 cm and is a derivative of the first branchial cleft. It receives sensory innervation primarily from cranial nerves V and X. Manipulation of the ear canal may produce a cough reflex (Arnold's reflex) in about 10 per cent of the population, and this is due to the stimulation of a branch of the vagus nerve. The external auditory canal is S-shaped, angulating backward and upward in the lateral

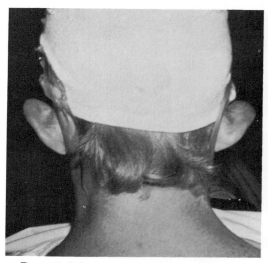

Figure 1–2. Back view of a patient with lop ears.

one third, with a forward and downward angulation in the medial two thirds. The lateral one third is cartilaginous, whereas the medial two thirds is bony. A slight narrowing exists at about the midportion of the external auditory canal (isthmus), and this makes removal of cerumen or foreign bodies deep in the canal a difficult task. Additionally, the skin of the bony canal is tightly adherent to the periosteum, causing extraordinary pain when the local tissues are traumatized or become inflamed. The skin of the cartilaginous canal is also firmly applied to the perichondrium and contains many small cerumen glands and hair follicles but is much less sensitive to touch.

The anterior canal wall is perforated by several small clefts known as the fissures of Santorini. These dehiscences permit the extension of inflammatory processes of the external auditory canal to the preauricular lymph nodes and parotid gland. This anatomic finding must be kept in mind when treating malignancies of the external auditory canal.

The external auditory canal not only serves as a conduit for sound energy but also acts as a tube resonator, with a definite resonant peak of approximately 12 dB in the vicinity of 3000 to 4000 Hz, and measurably enhances signals in the 2000 to 6000 Hz range. Because of its oblique course and the sensitive nature of the skin lining the canal, the external auditory canal also affords a measure of protection for the tympanic membrane and other middle ear structures.

Middle Ear

The tympanic cavity (middle ear) is the space medial to the tympanic membrane and lateral to the osseous labyrinth. It is approximately 15-mm high, 15-mm wide, and 2- to 6-mm deep. The portion of the cavity that extends above the tympanic membrane is called the epitympanum, and that which extends below the drumhead is known as the hypotympanum. The middle ear contains two muscles and three small bones, or ossicles, that conduct the sound energy to the oval window of the cochlea. The middle ear is derived embryologically from the first branchial pouch. The middle ear is not a closed cavity because it communicates posteriorly with the mastoid air cells and anteriorly with the nasopharynx through the eustachian tube (auditory tube) (Fig. 1–3).

Most of the lateral wall of the middle ear is limited by the tympanic membrane. The roof (tegmen tympani) is a thin plate of bone separating the middle ear from the middle cranial fossa. The petrosquamous suture (junction of the petrous and squamous portions of the temporal bone) crosses the tegmen tympani. This structure is not yet ossified in children and may allow direct passage of infection from the middle ear to the meninges of the middle cranial fossa. On occasion, adults have veins that pass through this suture to terminate in the venous sinuses within the skull. The suture and its component veins constitute a potential route for spread of middle ear infections to the meninges or venous sinuses or both. They are also a possible locus for spontaneous cerebral spinal fluid leakage.

The middle ear is lined by a mucous membrane (mucoperiosteum) in its entirety. This lining is continuous with that of mastoid air cells posteriorly and that of the eustachian tube anteriorly. The mucoperiosteum completely envelops the three ossicles

Figure 1–3. Diagram of middle ear system.

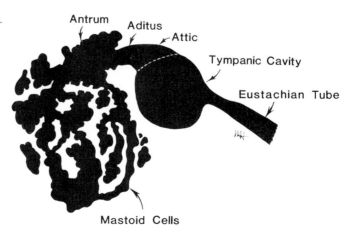

Antrum Aditus Attic Tympanic Cavity Eustachian Tube Mastoid Cells

within the middle ear. This mucous membrane is formed by an epithelium, a connective tissue layer, and the periosteum that covers the underlying bone. The epithelium is largely, although not solely, a respiratory epithelium.

Important structures adjacent to the middle ear that are usually separated from the cavity by a bony wall include the jugular foramen inferiorly, the carotid artery anteriorly and inferiorly, the inner ear medially, the middle cranial fossa superiorly, and the facial nerve paramedially and posteriorly.

Thirty per cent of people have air cells in the petrous portion of the temporal bone that are in communication with the middle ear. The petrous tip is anatomically near cranial nerves V and VI so that an inflammatory process of the middle ear can involve both of these cranial nerves by continuity, resulting in severe pain and paralysis of the ipsilateral lateral rectus muscle (Gradenigo's syndrome).

The three auditory ossicles (malleus, incus, and stapes) (Fig. 1–4) are contained in the middle ear. They are mobile and suspended by five ligaments (superior, lateral, and anterior malleal, posterior incudal, and oval window annular), two muscles, three

articulations (malleus to incus to stapes, and stapes to bony labyrinth), and the attachment of the malleus to the drumhead. The malleus is approximately 9-mm long and weighs about 23 mg. The incus is about 8 mm long and weighs about 27 mg; the stapes, the smallest ossicle, measures about 3 mm in height and weighs about 2.5 mg (Fig. 1–5).

The incudomalleal and incudostapedial joints are true diarthrodial joints (movable articulations with a synovial lining) and are therefore subject to fixation by systemic disease states that involve such joints. The articulation of the stapes with the osseous labyrinth is maintained by a fibrous anulus.

The eustachian tube opening is located anteriorly in the middle ear. At birth, the eustachian tube lies in the horizontal plane but, with growth, it becomes inclined to an angle of 40 to 45 degrees. According to many authors, this anatomic characteristic is accountable for the increased frequency of otitis media in the early years. The tube is not at the lowest level of the middle ear; therefore it does not function as a passive drain. The eustachian tube is usually closed and opens during deglutition as a result of the action of the tensor veli palatini muscle.

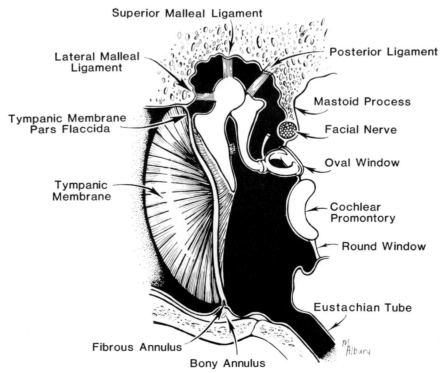

Figure 1–4. Diagram of coronal view of the middle ear.

of pressure between the middle ear and ambient air.

The tympanic membrane forms a semi-transparent partition between the external auditory canal and the middle ear cleft (Fig. 1–6). It has an elliptical configuration, measuring 9 to 10 mm vertically and 8 to 9 mm horizontally, with a concave outer surface. The deepest portion of the tympanic membrane concavity is located where the membrane is adherent to the umbo of the malleus. The most prominent feature on the lateral surface of the drumhead is the short process of the malleus. Alterations in the appearance of this structure can indicate middle ear effusion. Malleolar ligaments (anterior and posterior), which run from the short process to the anulus, mark the boundary of the pars tensa and pars flaccida. The pars flaccida plays an important role in the development of primary acquired cholesteatoma (see Chapter 3). When examining the normal drumhead, the physician sees a triangular light reflex extending from the umbo antero-inferiorly, representing the light reflected off the concave surface of the membrane.

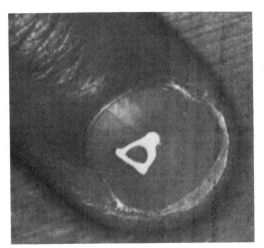

Figure 1–5. Human stapes on a fingernail.

Three main functions have been attributed to the eustachian tube: mucociliary clearance of fluids and/or particles from the middle ear to the nasopharynx, impedance of substances ascending from the nasopharynx toward the middle ear, and the equalization

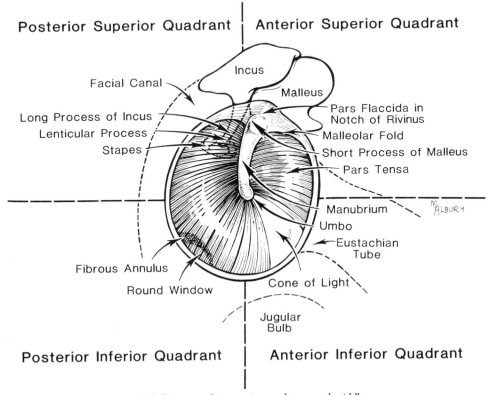

Figure 1–6. Diagram of tympanic membrane and middle ear.

The average thickness of the tympanic membrane is 0.074 mm and it weighs approximately 14 mg. The pars tensa is composed of three distinct layers: a lateral epidermis, which is a cornified squamous epithelium; a middle layer or lamina propria, with outer radial and inner circular collagenous fibers; and a medial mucosa, which is one cell layer thick. The pars flaccida, which is thicker than the pars tensa, is also composed of a lateral cornified squamous epithelium, a lamina propria, and a medial mucosal layer. The collagen and elastic fibers of the lamina propria are more irregular than those of the pars tensa, accounting, at least in part, for the thinner appearance of the pars flaccida. Retraction and invagination of a portion of this structure or a perforation can lead to cholesteatoma formation (see Chapter 3).

Three nerves pass through the middle ear. As previously noted, the facial nerve usually runs in a bony canal (fallopian canal) along the medial wall of the middle ear above the stapes and oval window. Frequently, however, dehiscences are present in the bony canal, which makes the nerve subject to surgical trauma and inflammation secondary to middle ear infection. Posterior to the oval window, the facial nerve turns to run inferiorly in the posterior wall of the middle ear, exiting the skull at the stylomastoid foramen.

Four types of nerve fibers travel with the facial nerve. General somatic afferent fibers supply the sensations of pain, temperature, and touch to the posterior superior external auditory canal, and general visceral efferent fibers supply parasympathetic innervation to the lacrimal gland, nose, and salivary glands (submandibular sublingual). Special visceral afferent fibers deliver the sensation of taste from the anterior two thirds of the tongue, and special visceral efferent fibers supply motor innervation to muscles of branchiogenic origin.

The second nerve that passes through the middle ear is the chorda tympani, a branch of the facial nerve. It leaves the facial nerve approximately 6 mm proximal to the stylomastoid foramen and enters the middle ear through a foramen on the posterior wall (iter chordae posterius). The chorda tympani nerve passes lateral to the long process of the incus and medial to the handle of the malleus, exiting the tympanic cavity anteriorly through a second bony foramen (canal of Huguier). It provides the sensation of taste to the anterior two thirds of the tongue and carries parasympathetic preganglionic fibers to the submandibular and sublingual glands. Lastly, Jacobson's nerve courses vertically over the promontory, carrying parasympathetic fibers from the interior salvatory nucleus to the parotid gland. Jacobson's nerve may be found immediately under the middle ear mucoperiosteum or in a bony canal. Glomus bodies can be identified in the middle ear, especially. These glomus bodies are of neural crest origin, serve as chemoreceptors, and occasionally undergo neoplastic transformation (glomus tympanicum, glomus jugulare).

The medial wall of the middle ear contains three additional important anatomic landmarks: the oval and round windows and the promontory. The oval window is normally occupied by the footplate of the stapes, has a surface area of about 3.5 mm^2, and is located in the posterior-superior quadrant of the medial wall. The round window is located several millimeters inferior to the oval window and lies in a plane perpendicular to that window. It lies beneath a bony ledge and has a surface area of approximately 2 mm^2. The round window functions as a pressure release for movement of inner ear fluids originating at the oval window. The promontory is a bony prominence anterior to both the round and oval windows. It represents the otic capsule lateral to the basal turn of the cochlea.

As previously noted, the most lateral ossicle, the malleus, is attached on one side to the tympanic membrane and on the other side to the second ossicle, the incus. The incus in turn articulates with the most medial of the ossicles, the stapes (Fig. 1–7).

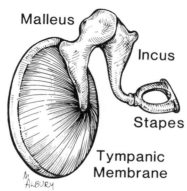

Figure 1–7. Diagram showing relationship between the tympanic membrane and the middle ear ossicles.

The footplate of the stapes rests in the oval window of the cochlea. Motion of the tympanic membrane is transmitted through the ossicular chain to the oval window and the cochlear fluids (perilymph and endolymph). A basic acoustic principle is that sound waves traveling in one medium will not easily transfer into another of different density. The middle ear, therefore, must act as an impedance-matching mechanism to increase the efficiency of sound energy transfer from a gaseous medium to a fluid medium. The characteristic acoustic impedance of air is 40 dynes per cm³. The acoustic impedance of the cochlear fluids is approximately equal to that of sea water, 160,000 dynes per cm³. Without an impedance-matching system, as much as 99.9 per cent of the acoustic energy at the air-cochlear interface would be reflected and only 0.1 per cent transmitted as an effective stimulus. This would represent approximately a 30-dB diminution in signal energy.

As part of the impedance mechanism, the concave conical configuration of the tympanic membrane improves sound transmission by minimizing distortion and enlarging the frequency response range. Most of the middle ear amplification, however, is derived from the hydraulic action of the oval window and tympanic membrane. The tympanic membrane has an effective surface area of approximately 55 mm², whereas the surface of the stapes footplate is 3.2 to 3.5 mm². Thus, the relatively large but weak excursions of the drumhead are converted to smaller but more forceful motions at the oval window. The mechanical lever effect of the ossicular chain adds additional imped-

ance matching by producing an amplification factor of about 1.3 to 1. This is due to the longer length of the malleus manipulating the shorter incus. The combined hydraulic and lever actions of the ossicles multiply the force of sound striking the tympanic membrane approximately 27 times, overcoming much of the resistance or impedance at the middle ear/inner ear interface (Fig. 1–8). As previously mentioned, the round window plays a critical role in auditory function, serving as a pressure relief area so that the steps can move the incompressible inner ear fluids when force is applied to the footplate.

In addition to its role in impedance matching, the tympanic membrane effectively seals the middle ear space from the external environment. This seal prevents sound waves from striking both the round and oval windows simultaneously, which would eliminate the necessary phase difference that occurs between these two windows. If this phase difference did not exist, sound waves would be propagated from both ends of the inner ear, and the waves would tend to cancel each other. This could produce up to a 20-dB hearing loss.

The maximum conductive hearing loss resulting from a total perforation of the pars tensa is about 40 to 45 dB. This loss is due to a decrease in hydraulic action and a loss of the phase difference at the round and oval windows. Smaller perforations have less effect, and the severity of the hearing loss depends upon the size and location of the perforation. Ossicular discontinuity or fixation with intact tympanic membrane may produce a 50- to 60-dB conductive hearing

Figure 1–8. Hydraulic action of the tympanic membrane and stapes.

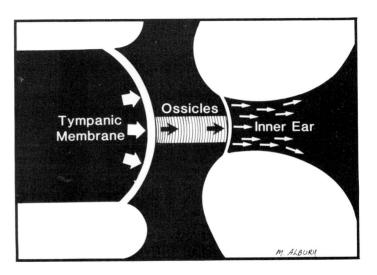

loss. Any increase in mass of the drumhead or ossicles produces a high-frequency hearing loss, whereas any increase in stiffness, as seen in early otosclerosis, produces a low-frequency conductive hearing loss.

The two muscles present in the middle ear are the tensor tympani muscle and the stapedius muscle. The tensor muscle of the tympanum is about 2-cm long and lies along the superiomedial aspect of the eustachian tube and the middle ear. At the cochleariform process, this muscle turns laterally and its tendon extends across the middle ear, inserting on the neck of the malleus. This muscle is of first branchial arch origin and, therefore, it is innervated by the fifth cranial nerve. The stapedius muscle is normally encased in a bony prominence (the pyramidal process) on the posterior wall of the middle ear. Its tendon attaches to the capitulum of the stapes, and because of its second branchial arch origin, it is innervated by the facial nerve. Although the exact function of the middle ear muscles is not known, both the stapedius muscle and the tensor muscle of the tympanum contract in the presence of loud auditory stimuli, reducing the motion of the ossicles. It is theorized that this re-

duction prevents harmful stimuli from entering the inner ear.

Inner Ear

The inner ear consists of three parts: the pars superior, which includes the utricle and semicircular canals; the pars inferior, which includes the saccule and cochlea; and the pars intermedia, which includes the endolymphatic duct and endolymphatic sac. The pars superior and pars intermedia will be discussed in Chapter 7. The cochlea of the pars inferior acts as a transducer to convert mechanical energy in the cochlear fluids to neural energy coded for frequency discrimination and intensity recognition. In man, the cochlea is a small coiled tube of approximately two and one-half turns and about 3.5-cm long. Visualized in cross section (Fig. 1–9), two membranes divide its interior into three chambers. The two larger chambers, the scala vestibuli and the scala tympani, contain perilymph, which has an electrolyte composition similar to extracellular fluid. The scala vestibuli is sealed at one end by the stapes footplate in the oval window and the scala tympani is sealed at the base of the cochlea by the round window membrane. At

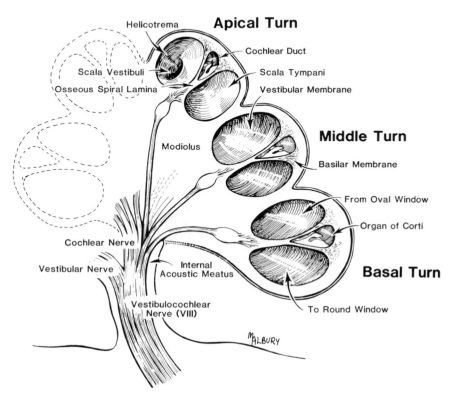

Figure 1–9. Cross section of the cochlea.

the apex of the cochlea, the scala vestibuli and scala tympani communicate by way of a small opening, the helicotrema.

The cochlear duct, or scala media, is triangular in cross section and forms the smallest of the inner ear partitions. It is separated from the scala vestibuli by Reissner's membrane and from the scala tympani by the basilar membrane. The lateral wall is primarily composed of the stria vascularis and spiral prominence. The scala media contains endolymph, which resembles intracellular fluid in its electrolyte composition. Within the scala media is the organ of Corti, which sits on the basilar membrane (the partition between the scala media and the scala tympani). Liberally speaking, the organ of Corti is composed of inner and outer hair cells, inner phalangeal and outer phalangeal (Deiter's) cells, inner and outer pillar cells, Hensen's cells, Claudius' cells, and inner sulcus cells. In the organ of Corti, receptor elements (hair cells) are arranged in three outer rows containing about 12,500 hair cells and one inner row containing about 3500 hair cells. Sitting atop the stereocilea of the hair cells is the tectorial membrane. This structure projects from the spiral limbus and is presumably formed by the interdental cells or Huschke's teeth cells of that structure. The tectorial membrane is made up of a gelatinous mucopolysaccharide ground substance containing keratin-like fibrils. It is attached to the inner phalangeal cells in the area of Hensen's stripe and again, at its margin, near the most lateral Deiter's cells of Hensen's cells.

Vibrations of the cochlear fluids induced by stapes motion differentially distort the basilar membrane. The maximum point of basilar membrane displacement is frequency dependent, with higher frequencies represented at the cochlear base, where the basilar membrane is narrow (approximately 80 μ) and stiff; and lower frequencies represented near the apex, where the basilar membrane is relatively wider (500 μ) and more compliant. This displacement of the basilar membrane results in a shearing force between the tectorial membrane and the stereocilea of the receptor hair cells, resulting in alteration of membrane potentials and ultimately in the depolarization of the hair cells. Locally weighted receptor potentials that result from this depolarization can be detected and measured and are known as cochlear microphonics. These alternating current potentials reflect hair cell activity,

faithfully reproduce acoustic signals, and reflect the waveform of vibration of the cochlear partition without latency, refractory period, adaptation, or fatigue. Cochlear microphonics can be used to assess receptor integrity and, when used as a part of the technique known as electrocochleography, permit an objective measurement of peripheral auditory function. This technique can also assist in the differentiation of cochlear sensory hearing loss and neural or retrocochlear hearing loss. The nature of the fluid under the tectorial membrane and that which is in contact with the pillar cells (Corti's duct) and hair cells (spaces of Neul) is of physiologic importance. It appears to resemble perilymph in its electrolyte composition. This fluid may simply be perilymph from the scala tympani that has passed through the habenula perforatae (perforations in the bony spiral lamina through which the nerve fibers to the hair cells pass). Investigation continues actively in this area because the understanding of inner ear fluid homeostasis is paramount to understanding the pathophysiology of many auditory vestibular disorders.

The remaining structures of the organ of Corti are quite poorly understood. The phalangeal cells and pillar cells are, in conjunction with the reticular lamina, primarily responsible for supporting the architecture of the organ of Corti, but recent evidence suggests that they may also play a role in fluid transport. Hensen's cells store lipids. It has also been proposed that they supply nutrients for outer hair cells and Deiter's cells as part of their function. The functions proposed for inner sulcus cells, Claudius' cells, and external sulcus cells are similar. These functions have not been proved but include fluid transport and, perhaps, removal of particulate matter from the endolymph. The lateral wall of the cochlea is composed of the stria vascularis, the spiral ligament, and the spiral prominence. The stria vascularis consists of three cell types. Marginal or chromophil (dark) cells line the endolymphatic surface, with short microvilli projecting into the scala media. They are joined by tight junctions. Fluid transport has been proposed as a function of these marginal cells but it has not been proved. Intermediate or chromophobe (light) cells are irregular and stellate shaped; they interdigitate with the marginal cells. Their function is not known. The basal cells, like the marginal cells, are connected by tight junctions. They lie adjacent to capillaries of the spiral ligament. Their function is also poorly understood. The stria vascularis has a high metabolic rate and, as a unit, is thought to be at least partially responsible for maintaining the endolymphatic direct current potential and homeostasis. The spiral prominence lies just inferior to the stria vascularis. Flattened cuboidal cells that cover connective tissue and capillaries line the endolymphatic space. The function of the spiral prominence remains unknown. The spiral ligament lies behind the stria vascularis and extends from the scala vestibuli to the scala tympani. Its architecture consists of many keratin fibrils in a loose meshwork, with multiple capillaries. As with many other areas in the organ of Corti, inner ear fluid balance is believed to be influenced by this structure but this has not been proved.

Reissner's membrane, the partition between the scala vestibuli and scala media, is two cell layers thick. The cells on the scala media side are bridged by tight junctions and have microvilli projecting into the endolymph. The cells on the scala vestibuli side lack tight junctions and microvilli. It has been proposed that Reissner's membrane is selectively permeable, allowing certain ions to pass while impeding others. The auditory nerve is a connecting link between the peripheral auditory mechanism and the central processing centers. Neural impulses generated by the receptor elements are transmitted by approximately 30,000 afferent neural fibers of the auditory division of the eighth cranial nerve. The cell bodies of the first order neurons of the acoustic nerve are all contained in the spiral ganglion. Ninety-five per cent of all afferent nerve fibers originate on inner hair cells, whereas the remainder originate on outer hair cells. The auditory nerve also delivers efferent fibers, by way of the olivocochlear bundle, to both inner and outer hair cells. Although few in number (about 500 neurons), these efferent fibers are widely distributed through an enormous branching system. The function of the efferent system is not well understood, but it is believed to exert a type of modulation or feedback effect on the afferent system.

Preliminary Discussion and Classification of Hearing Loss

The ear manifests its disorders in a limited number of ways. Hearing loss is, as men-tioned previously, a sign or symptom; it may occur alone, as part of a more generalized disease process, or as one manifestation of a syndrome. Other symptoms that may accompany hearing loss include noises or ringing in the ears (tinnitus), dizziness, unsteadiness, or vertigo, pain in the ear (otalgia), aural fullness, and drainage from the ear (otorrhea). Any of these symptoms may lead the patient with auditory dysfunction to seek treatment. It is helpful to understand the significance and origin of each of these symptoms.

The problem of noises, ringing, or buzzing in the ears (tinnitus) may be subjective or objective. Subjective tinnitus is by far the more common type and is usually thought to arise as a manifestation of damage or injury to the cochlea or the auditory nerve. Objective tinnitus (tinnitus that can be documented by others) is less common and usually represents a local vascular disorder. Tinnitus will be discussed in depth in Chapter 6.

Contiguous to the auditory portion of the ear is the developmentally older and, therefore, more resilient portion known as the vestibular apparatus or vestibular labyrinth. Together with the visual and kinesthetic sensory systems, the vestibular system is responsible for the maintenance of equilibrium and spatial positioning. Since the sensory receptors of the vestibular system and auditory system are quite similar in type and function and share a common fluid, it is not illogical that disorders of one system might be shared with the other. Thus the presence of vestibular dysfunction (vertigo) may accompany auditory dysfunction. Pain in the ear (otalgia), aural fullness, and drainage from the ear (otorrhea) usually suggest local inflammatory problems. Although the vestibular labyrinth is closely related to the cochlea from an anatomic standpoint, its anatomy and physiology have been described in Chapter 7 because of the association between the vestibular labyrinth and vertigo.

Clinical and audiologic evaluations reveal several factors useful in the classification and understanding of hearing loss. First and perhaps most important, the hearing loss is classified as conductive, sensorineural, or mixed. A conductive hearing loss results from a malfunction in the gathering of sound by the external ear, secondary to obstruction of the external auditory canal, or incomplete or inefficient transfer of sound energy to the cochlea by the eardrum or the ossicles of the middle ear. It is often possible to improve conductive hearing losses surgically. Sensorineural hearing loss may be caused by a lesion of the sensory receptor elements in the cochlea or the auditory nerve (peripheral sensorineural hearing loss) or a lesion of the higher processing centers (central sensorineural hearing loss). Cochlear hearing loss is a primary failure of the receptor or transducer mechanisms within the cochlea. Retrocochlear hearing loss indicates a failure of the auditory nerve or central processing areas. The clinical differentiation of these types of hearing loss can be made by physical examination and specialized audiologic testing (see Chapters 4 and 8). Retrocochlear hearing loss may frequently be associated with the presence of an intracranial neoplasm. The possibility of such a neoplasm being present must be eliminated in every case of retrocochlear hearing loss. Sensorineural hearing losses are usually not reversed by surgery.

Mixed hearing losses are those that have elements of both conductive and sensorineural disorders. Other characteristics of hearing loss also aid in classification. A hearing loss may be present at birth (congenital) or delayed in onset, genetic or nongenetic, or progressive, stable, or sudden. Accurate classification can be a significant aid in the evaluation of a given case of hearing loss. Overlap between classifications is necessary owing to the variable manifestations of several syndromes (Tables 1–2 to 1–9).

CONGENITAL CONDUCTIVE AND MIXED HEARING LOSS

Congenital hearing loss that is conductive or that combines conductive and sensorineural components may occur alone or as part of a syndrome and may or may not be transmitted genetically. Attention is directed to early diagnosis and treatment. Treatment is surgical when possible and early habilitation is imperative. Medical management alone is not adequate, although simple middle ear effusion and rare cases of congenital hypothyroidism may respond to medical therapy. Assessment of associated anomalies, genetic and psychosocial counseling, and epidemiologic study may be appropriate. Tables 1–2 and 1–3 lists the causes of congenital conductive and mixed hearing loss. These hearing losses will be discussed in Chapter 2.

DELAYED CONDUCTIVE AND MIXED HEARING LOSS

Genetic as well as nongenetic factors may contribute to delayed conductive or mixed hearing loss. Treatment of these conditions

Table 1–2. GENETIC CAUSES OF CONGENITAL CONDUCTIVE AND MIXED HEARING LOSS

Cause	Mode of Inheritance	Manifestations
Treacher Collins syndrome	Dominant	External auditory canal atresia Middle ear anomalies Downward slanting eyes Lower lid coloboma Flat malar eminence Micrognathia
Apert's syndrome	Dominant	Frontal bossing Exophthalmos Hypoplastic maxilla Syndactyly
Marfan's syndrome	Dominant	Pigeon breast Dolichoecephaly Hammer toes
Pierre Robin syndrome	Dominant	Glossoptosis Micrognathia Cleft palate
Crouzon's syndrome	Dominant	Premature fusion of cranial sutures Shallow orbits Exophthalmos Parrot nose Hypoplastic maxilla
Fanconi's syndrome	Recessive	Abnormal or missing thumbs Mental retardation Pancytopenia Skeletal, heart, and renal malformations

Table 1–3. NONGENETIC CAUSES OF CONGENITAL CONDUCTIVE AND MIXED HEARING LOSS

Viral infection (e.g., rubella)
Ototoxic drugs (e.g., thalidomide)
Metabolic disorders (e.g., hypothyroidism)
Canal stenosis
Congenital cholesteatoma
Cretinism
Middle ear effusion

is usually surgical, although medical therapy works well under some circumstances. Otitis media, for example, is a very frequent cause of conductive hearing loss that may, depending upon its etiology, require medical, surgical, or combined therapy. The causes of delayed conductive and mixed hearing loss are shown in Tables 1–4 and 1–5. These hearing losses will be further discussed in Chapter 2.

CONGENITAL SENSORINEURAL HEARING LOSS

The most important factors in any congenital hearing loss, whether sensorineural, conductive, or mixed, are early diagnosis and treatment. At the present time, medical and surgical treatments have little effect on primary sensorineural hearing loss. Possible contributory mechanisms, however, should be vigorously pursued and treated. Treatment should be directed toward early habilitation and genetic and social counseling. The genetic and nongenetic disorders responsible for congenital sensorineural hearing loss are shown in Tables 1–6 and 1–7. This type of hearing loss will be further discussed in Chapter 4.

DELAYED SENSORINEURAL HEARING LOSS

Tables 1–8 and 1–9 list the causes of delayed sensorineural hearing loss. Delayed genetic and nongenetic sensorineural hearing losses are, with a few exceptions, not amenable to medical or surgical therapy. Hearing losses resulting from metabolic derangements, Meniere's disease, neurosyphilis, or space-occupying lesions can often be effectively treated by various medical and surgical techniques. Again, rehabilitation, counseling, and epidemiologic study are important considerations in the management of these cases. Delayed sensorineural hearing loss will be discussed further in Chapter 4.

Table 1–4. GENETIC CAUSES OF DELAYED CONDUCTIVE AND MIXED HEARING LOSS

Cause	Mode of Inheritance	Manifestations
Albers-Schönberg disease	Recessive	Osteopetrosis, with brittle sclerotic bones
		Cranial neuropathies
		Large skull and mandible
		Bone marrow obliteration
Engelmann's disease	Dominant	Diaphyseal dysplasia
Hurler's syndrome	Recessive	Abnormal deposition of mucopolysaccharides
		Frontal bossing
		Stubby digits
		Mental retardation
		Hepatosplenomegaly
Otosclerosis	Dominant	Bone resorption and redeposition
		Progressive bilateral involvement
		Onset in third or fourth decade
Rheumatoid Arthritis	Variable	Multiple joint involvement with pain, inflammation, and limited motion
Osteogenesis imperfecta	Uncertain	Fragile bones
		Large skull
		Blue sclera
		Triangular facies
		Hemorrhagic tendencies
		Stapes fixation
Paget's disease	Dominant	Osteitis deformans, with deformities of skull and long bones
		Cranial neuropathies

Table 1–5. NONGENETIC CAUSES OF DELAYED CONDUCTIVE AND MIXED HEARING LOSS

Presenting Cause	Underlying Cause
Otitis media	
Acute infectious	Allergy
	Bacteria
	Virus
Chronic	Cholesteatoma
	Osteitis
	Structural abnormality
Luetic	Syphilis
Serous	Allergy
	Regional infection (e.g., sinus, nasopharynx)
	Immunoglobulin deficiency
	Metabolic disturbance
	Previous irradiation therapy
	Mechanical obstruction of eustachian tube orifice
	Interference with eustachian tube lymphatic drainage
	Neuromuscular abnormalities (e.g., cleft palate)
	Polyarteritis nodosa
	Wegner's granulomatosis
	Eosinophilic granuloma
	Neoplasm
Tuberculous	Tuberculosis
Trauma	Tympanic membrane rupture and ossicular discontinuity
Tumor	Obstruction of the external canal and middle ear

Table 1–7. NONGENETIC CAUSES OF CONGENITAL SENSORINEURAL HEARING LOSS

Environmental Factors

Intrauterine Factors
  Infection
  Ototoxic drugs
  Metabolic disorders
  Irradiation

Perinatal Insults
  Erythroblastosis fetalis
  Trauma
  Anoxia
  Prematurity

SUDDEN SENSORINEURAL HEARING LOSS

Sudden sensorineural hearing loss, complete or incomplete, unilateral or bilateral, is a true medical emergency because treatment success varies inversely with the time interval between symptoms and onset of therapy. Treatment that is begun later than 2 weeks following the onset of sudden sensorineural hearing loss is usually of no value. Proposed treatment is directed toward

Table 1–6. GENETIC CAUSES OF CONGENITAL SENSORINEURAL HEARING LOSS*

Cause	Mode of Inheritance	Manifestations
Temporal bone deformities	Usually dominant	Michel's total aplasia
		Partial aplasias of Mondini, Scheibe, and Alexander
Pendred's syndrome	Recessive	Coexistent nonendemic goiter
		Greatest hearing loss at high frequencies
		Unresponsive to thyroid extract
Jervell and Lange-Nielsen syndrome	Recessive	Prolonged Q–T interval on electrocardiogram (EKG)
		Profound sensorineural hearing loss
		Frequent syncope
		Possible sudden death
Waardenburg's syndrome	Dominant	Lateral displacement of medial canthi
		White forelock
		Heterochromia iridis
		Hypoplasia of the nasal alae
Usher's syndrome	Recessive	Progressive retinitis pigmentosa
Leopard syndrome	Dominant	Lentigenes
		EKG abnormalities
		Pulmonary stenosis
		Abnormalities of the genitalia
		Retardation of growth

*From Meyerhoff, W. L.: Diagnostic protocol for deafness in medical management. Laryngoscope 88:960–973, 1978. Reproduced with permission.

Table 1–8. GENETIC CAUSES OF DELAYED SENSORINEURAL HEARING LOSS

Cause	Mode of Inheritance	Manifestations
Progressive familial sensorineural hearing loss	Dominant, recessive, or X-linked	Early or late onset Isolated entity or part of syndrome
Alport's syndrome	Dominant	Progressive hearing loss, becoming manifest by about age 10 years Glomerulonephritis Refractory to treatment
Alstrom's syndrome	Recessive	Nystagmus and visual loss secondary to retinal degeneration at about age 1 year Progressive hearing loss just prior to adolescence Diabetes mellitus shortly after adolescence
Refsum's syndrome	Recessive	Onset in second decade Visual loss secondary to retinitis pigmentosa Ataxia Muscle wasting Ichthyosis
Friedreich's ataxia	Recessive	Nystagmus Optic atrophy Ataxia
von Recklinghausen's disease	Dominant	Acoustic neuroma formation Ataxia Visual loss Involvement of cranial nerves V through X Café-au-lait spots
Primary amyloidosis	Dominant	Systemic amyloid infiltration

the contributing factors and maximizing the environment for recovery. Sudden sensorineural hearing loss will be covered in depth in Chapter 5.

Table 1–9. NONGENETIC CAUSES OF DELAYED SENSORINEURAL HEARING LOSS

Noise

Head trauma
  Temporal bone fracture
  Labyrinthine concussion

Sudden pressure change
  Environmental
  Cerebrospinal fluid

Metabolic disturbances
  Hypothyroidism
  Abnormal glucose tolerance
  Adrenopituitary disorders
  Hyperlipoproteinemia
  Chronic renal disease
  Hyperparathyroidism

Toxic substances
  Heavy metals (e.g., lead, mercury)
  Antibiotics (e.g., aminoglycosides)
  Diuretics (e.g., ethacrynic acid, furosemide)
  Aspirin
  Cigarettes
  Toxins of typhoid fever and diphtheria

Space-occupying lesions in cerebellopontine angle
  Acoustic neuromas
  Meningiomas
  Vascular anomalies
  Congenital cholesteatoma

Inflammatory disease
  Viral infection (e.g., measles, mumps, adenovirus type III, herpesvirus)
  Bacterial infection (e.g., meningococcal meningitis, suppurative labyrinthitis)
  Neurosyphilis
  Allergic inflammation

Meniere's disease

Whatever the classification or associated symptomatology, the simple documentation of a hearing impairment is not sufficient. Every effort should be made to understand the cause of the disorder and its implications for the impaired individual.

General Diagnosis

Hearing impairment is a medical problem and, as such, a firm medical diagnosis is required before treatment and rehabilitation are begun. This may, at times, be just a reasonable working diagnosis while more clues are sought. All too often, the underlying process is ignored while the symptoms of auditory dysfunction are described and categorized and the patient empirically treated, or worse yet, informed that nothing can be done. The terms presbycusis and noise-induced hearing loss are frequently too easily and incorrectly used when further investigation is warranted. The primary aim of the medical investigation is to consider all possible causes, intrinsic (genetic) as well as extrinsic (e.g., metabolic, inflammatory, drug related, tumors, trauma, neurologic disease). Often several factors may contribute to the loss of auditory function, and one must be careful to look for every possible etiology (Table 1–10).

MEDICAL HISTORY

A diagnostic protocol for the evaluation of hearing loss is provided in Table 1–10. A good medical history should be the first step in any patient evaluation. Failure to take an adequate history is the most common error made in evaluating the patient with hearing loss. The diagnosis may be obvious from the history alone.

It is important to ascertain whether the hearing loss is unilateral or bilateral for diagnostic and therapeutic reasons. The mode of onset and rate of progression (sudden, insidious) also have important implications (see Chapter 5). The age at which the hearing loss occurred will help to direct the questioning, since certain conditions are unique to the young whereas others are unique to the elderly. In the evaluation of a patient with congenital hearing loss, for example, a perinatal history, including questions regarding the pregnancy, delivery, and early postpartum period, must be obtained. The importance of determining the presence of maternal infection (e.g., rubella), irradiation, metabolic disorders (e.g., hypothyroidism) or medications (e.g., thalidomide, aminoglycosides) cannot be exaggerated. Similarly, one must inquire about a difficult and prolonged delivery, the use of medications, and the occurrence of neonatal anoxia, trauma, or jaundice. Of equal importance in the evaluation of a patient with congenital hearing loss is the recognition of associated nonaural abnormalities that might suggest a syndrome (e.g., Treacher Collins syndrome, Apert's syndrome, Crouzon's syndrome, Fanconi's syndrome).

A thorough family history is also important in the evaluation of every patient with hearing loss in an effort to identify familial hearing loss or familial diseases that may be associated with hearing loss (Tables 1–2 to 1–9). In some instances the patient is advised to see a geneticist in order to obtain accurate genetic counseling.

Additional questions should be asked relating to the complaints of otorrhea, otalgia, tinnitus, vertigo, visual or gait disturbances, aural fullness, diplacusis, or recruitment. Symptoms associated with hearing loss may be of diagnostic value. The presence of vertigo suggests a lesion involving the vestibular system as well as the auditory system, whereas otorrhea suggests infection. The presence of otalgia suggests the presence of infection, a foreign body, or neoplasm. This symptom might be misleading, however, since in about 50 per cent of patients with otalgia, the pain originates from a site other than the ear (e.g., temporomandibular joint, cervical spine, hypopharynx). Tinnitus is a rather nonspecific symptom, whereas diplacusis and recruitment suggest a cochlear site of the lesion. Some symptom complexes (fluctuant hearing, incapacitating episodic vertigo, aural fullness, and tinnitus) are almost diagnostic.

Lastly, one must inquire about possible predisposing factors (e.g., noise exposure, ototoxic drugs) or precipitating events (e.g., head trauma) as well as signs or symptoms of conditions known to predispose the individual to hearing loss (e.g., hypothyroidism, multiple sclerosis, blood dyscrasias, arteriosclerosis, allergy, diabetes mellitus, congenital or acquired neurosyphilis, renal disease). In children too young to complain of hearing loss clues should be sought that might suggest a hearing loss problem (e.g., delayed speech development, inattention, sitting close to the television, pulling at the ears, or early personality problems).

PHYSICAL EXAMINATION

A comprehensive physical examination with emphasis on the neurotologic aspects of the head and neck is required when evaluating all cases of hearing loss. Abnormalities of the tympanic membrane or its mobility are associated with abnormalities of the impedance-matching mechanism and, therefore, hearing loss. When tympanic membrane perforation is present, the middle ear mucosa can be studied. The application of pressure to the external ear canal in the presence of the tympanic membrane perforation (fistula test) may result in the sensation of vertigo with nystagmus, suggesting communication between the middle ear and inner ear (e.g., cholesteatoma erosion into the horizontal semicircular canal). Hennebert's sign (positive fistula test with an intact tympanic membrane) is suggestive of neurosensory syphilis, Meniere's disease, or inner ear fistula.

Evaluation of all cranial nerves is part of a good neurotologic examination. A decreased corneal reflex, for example, may be due to pressure on cranial nerve V by an acoustic neuroma. External examination of the eye is important in the search for nystagmus and discolorations of the iris. Fundoscopic examination may reveal previously undetected nystagmus or retinal abnormalities, such as retinitis pigmentosa. In lesions in which increased intracranial pressure occurs, papilledema is identified. Additional changes in the optic disc, such as the temporal pallor of multiple sclerosis, may also be identified. Sometimes the physical examination alone makes the diagnosis obvious, as in Waardenburg's syndrome, in which the patient manifests white forelock, dystopic canthorum, and heterochromia iridis. A fairly good cranial nerve examination can be performed with minimal equipment. Olfaction can be tested, with the use of three small bottles, one containing coffee, one containing distilled water, and one containing ammonia. Eighty-five per cent of the normal population should recognize the smell of coffee. Failure to do so suggests anosmia. The distilled water should issue no smell, and the ammonia should irritate the nasal mucosa (cranial nerve V). A patient that claims to smell distilled water or denies sensation with inhaled ammonia is either confused or malingering.

The office nurse can check vision. Studying the extraocular movements will identify abnormalities of cranial nerves III, IV, and VI. Touching the forehead, cornea, and cheek with a wisp of cotton is a good test for cranial nerve V and studying the muscles of expression will detect a lesion of cranial nerve VIII. Cranial nerve VIII can be tested with tuning forks for hearing and the Romberg test for balance. The cranial nerves IX and X are responsible for the gag reflex, whereas cranial nerve X is totally responsible for the motor innervation of the vocal cords. Cranial nerve XI can be tested by having the patient shrug the shoulders or turn the head against force. Tongue motion is governed by cranial nerve XII.

Careful visual inspection of the auricle, external auditory canal, and tympanic membrane should be performed. A halogen otoscope provides excellent light and magnification for this procedure. A description of the normal tympanic membrane has already been provided. Variations in normalcy should be recorded. A pneumatic attachment to the otoscope can be used to assess tympanic membrane mobility. Slight to moderate mobility is normal. Turning fork tests are also of diagnostic help. They are based on the following physiologic facts: (1) The inner ear is normally twice as sensitive to sound conducted by air as opposed to that conducted by bone, and (2) in the presence of a purely conductive hearing loss, the involved ear is spared the input of environmental noise, making it more sensitive to sound conducted by bone.

The most clinical information can be gained by using tuning forks that naturally vibrate at 512 Hz, 1024 Hz, and 2048 Hz. Tuning forks that vibrate at lower frequencies provide a tactile stimulus, which often confuses results. Tactile stimulation may also occur if the tuning fork is struck too hard. All tests should be performed in a quiet room.

The Rinne tuning fork test compares the subject's ability to detect the tuning fork's vibrations in air with his ability to detect the tuning fork's vibration by direct bone conduction. In the Rinne test, the tuning fork is struck gently against the elbow to induce vibration and placed firmly against the mastoid process of the patient's ear (position 1). Once the patient is able to appreciate the sound level, the tuning fork is moved to a position just lateral to the external auditory canal, with its tines parallel to the direction of the auditory canal (position 2). The patient then judges whether the perceived sound was louder in position 1 or position 2. The Rinne test is considered to be positive if the subject hears normally (air conduction better than bone conduction) and negative if the patient hears abnormally (bone conduction better than air conduction). The Rinne will be positive in patients with normal hearing or with sensorineural hearing loss and will be negative in patients with a conductive hearing loss. Depending on the frequency, a negative Rinne indicates at least a 15-dB conductive hearing loss (Fig. 1–10).

In the Weber test, the vibrating tuning fork is placed firmly in the midline of the skull or mandible (Fig. 1–10). The patient reports localization of the sound to the right, left, or midline. The mechanical energy conducted through the bone will result in sound perceived as louder than normal in an ear with conductive hearing loss and quieter than normal in an ear with sensorineural hearing loss. Thus, in unilateral hearing loss, sound localized to the better hearing ear suggests a contralateral senorineural hearing loss whereas sound localized to the poorer hearing ear suggests an ipsilateral conductive hearing loss. Mixed hearing loss and com-

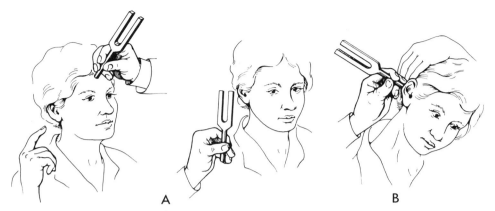

Figure 1–10. The Weber *(A)* and Rinne *(B)* tuning fork tests.

binations of hearing loss between the ears will provide a less exacting result.

The Bing test is used to verify the presence of a conductive hearing loss and to approximate the magnitude of the loss. The tuning fork is placed firmly over the mastoid cortex, and a conductive hearing loss is created by tightly occluding the external auditory meatus, using the index finger. In normal patients and in those patients with a sensorineural type of hearing loss, the perceived intensity of the tuning fork's signal will increase when the ear canal is blocked. However, in the patient with a marked conductive hearing loss, there will be no change in the signal's intensity when the canal is occluded. When the test is performed properly, an apparent diminution of signal strength when the canal is blocked is due either to confusion on the part of the patient or malingering. These simple tests can be of great benefit in determining the approximate magnitude of hearing loss and as a cross check of audiometric data (Table 1–10).

AUDIOMETRIC EXAMINATION AND LABORATORY TESTS

After the history and physical examination, an audiometric evaluation should be obtained to quantify the hearing loss and to serve as a baseline with which future studies can be compared. Special audiologic studies are included in the evaluation to establish the site of lesion in asymmetric hearing loss or to diagnose those cases of hearing loss without apparent cause (see Chapter 8). Laboratory and radiographic studies can be obtained as necessary to confirm or rule out possible etiologies. There are a multitude of

laboratory tests that may be indicated in the investigation of a sensorineural deafness, depending on the history and physical examination. These tests should not be ordered indiscriminately because the expense can mount rapidly. However, a disservice to the patient results from the failure to pursue appropriate diagnostic studies. Tests will be cost effective only if one carefully uses the history and physical examination as guides. Tests that evaluate endocrine function include the glucose tolerance test, thyroid function studies, and a variety of tests that investigate the pituitary-adrenal axis. The perchlorate or thiocyanate flush are diagnostic tests for Pendred's syndrome.

Abnormalities of renal function are found in Alport's syndrome, as these patients manifest proteinuria and hematuria secondary to glomerulonephritis. The blood urea nitrogen and creatinine clearance are also elevated in Alport's syndrome. Aminoaciduria occurs in a variety of syndromes associated with sensorineural hearing loss. Excessive mucopolysaccharide excretion occurs in Hurler's syndrome and the other mucopolysaccharidoses, whereas mannose-rich components occur in the urine of patients with mannosidoses. During aminoglycoside antibiotics therapy, to prevent overdosing, blood urea nitrogen levels and creatinine levels of the patient should be monitored, since these antibiotics are excreted in the urine.

Hematologic studies may also play an important role in the determination of the cause of sensorineural hearing loss. Both hypocoagulable states and hypercoagulable states are associated with hearing loss, and the investigation of these states includes tests of platelet function, prothrombin time,

Table 1–10. DIAGNOSTIC PROTOCOL FOR DEAFNESS

History

Otolaryngologic and complete general

Physical Examination

Otolaryngologic (head and neck and complete general, including cranial nerve assessment). Include
    Fundoscopic evaluation
    Neurologic evaluation, especially of the cranial nerves
    Medical evaluation for vascular, collagen, or other systemic diseases

Audiology

(Frequent re-evaluation will assess progression, improvement, or stability)
    Tuning fork tests—Rinne and Weber (others optional); use Bárány noise box when necessary. These are to be done
        by a physician to corroborate audiologic findings
    Whispered voice and shout test (using Bárány Masking)
    Pure tone air and bone
    Speech reception threshold
    Phonetic balance (discrimination)
    Modified tone decay test
    Loudness recruitment test (short increment sensitivity test [SIS] and/or Alternate Binaural Loudness Balance [ABLB])
    Békésy air conduction and audiogram
    Binaural pitch matching
    Impedance measurements to include acoustic reflex
    Other tests are indicated, such as difference limen for frequency (DLF), temporal integration, competing messages,
        Stenger tests, evoked response, etc.

Vestibular Evaluation

    Rhomberg, tandem standing gait
    Spontaneous nystagmus (direction and type)
    Positional test
    Caloric test (3 ml ice water to compare gross symmetry; 30 ml ice water to prove a dead labyrinth)
    Electronystagmography (using air caloric testing method)

X-Ray

    Skull
    Chest
    Mastoid and internal auditory meatus
    Polytomography of labyrinth and other parts of temporal bone as indicated
    Posterior fossa myelogram (clivogram) for suspected retrochochlear lesion
    Computerized axial tomography

Cardiac Evaluation

    Vital signs (blood pressure, pulse, respiration, temperature)
    Electrocardiogram

Laboratory Tests

Hematologic
    White blood count and differential
    Hemoglobin
    Sedimentation rate
    Platelet count

Coagulation
    Prothrombin consumption
    Prothrombin time
    Partial thromboplastic time (PTT)
    Platelet count
    Definitive studies if either hyper or hypocoagulation is suspected

Table 1–10. DIAGNOSTIC PROTOCOL FOR DEAFNESS (*Continued*)

Renal
  Urine analysis
  Blood urea nitrogen (BUN)
  Creatinine

Endocrine
  Thiocyanate flush (Pendred's syndrome)
  Fasting blood sugar (FBS)
  Adenocorticotropic (ACTH) plasma cortisol stimulation test
  Protein-bound iodine (PBI)
  Cholesterol and triglycerides
  Glucose tolerance test

Biochemical
  Total protein
  Albumin
  Globulin
Serum electrophoresis: Na, K, Ca, Cl, CO_2 (optional unless indicated by history or examination)

Liver Function
(optional unless indicated by history or examination)

Serologic and Immunologic
  Venereal Disease Research Laboratory (VDRL)
  Fluorescent treponemal antibody (FTA)
  Lupus erythematosus (LE) cell preparation
  Heterophil agglutinin titer

Lumbar Puncture
  Opening pressure
  Color
  Cell count and differential
  Protein (total and electrophoresis)
  Electrolytes
  Serology
  Glucose
  Viral culture
  Culture for bacteria, fungi, and acid-fast bacilli

*Viral Studies**
1. Acute specimens should be obtained as early as possible within, but not after, 21 days of the onset of deafness
   a. Whole clotted blood (for culture and titer)
   b. Stool
   c. Washings from throat or nasopharynx
   d. Cerebrospinal fluid
   e. Under special conditions such as when tympanotomy is performed to evaluate a perforated round window, fluid from the middle or inner ear may be available for viral culture. This should be inoculated into tissue culture in the operating room

2. Convalescent whole clotted blood for culture and titer should be obtained between the third and fifth week after the onset of deafness and at least 14 days after obtaining the acute whole clotted blood

3. Handling of specimens. Since viral organisms are fragile and poorly withstand storage or mailing, they are preferably hand-carried. Viral specimens should be labeled, in addition to identifying data, with "Special Study—Deafness"

Exploratory Tympanotomy
This procedure is indicated when spontaneous rupture of the round window or other middle ear pathology is suspected, or if perilymph is to be sampled for diagnostic purposes

*Contact your nearest or state virology laboratory for specific instructions regarding the handling of specimens.

partial thromboplastin time, thromboplastin reabsorption, and other more sophisticated studies of coagulation.

Lipoprotein levels are elevated in hyperlipoproteinemia and lipoprotein electrophoresis may be obtained if hyperlipoproteinemia is believed to be the cause of the hearing loss. The white cell count will be elevated in infection and occasionally in leukemias. In both these cases, sensorineural hearing loss may result. Serologic tests are important in the diagnosis of syphilis and both the Venereal Disease Research Laboratory (VDRL) and fluorescent treponemal antibody absorption tests (FTA-ABS) should be obtained. Rheumatoid factor and fluorescent antinuclear antibody (FANA) tests may indicate collagen diseases, and occasionally, a heterophil antibody test will indicate mononucleosis as the etiologic agent of the sensorineural hearing loss.

ROENTGENOGRAPHIC EXAMINATIONS

Roentgenography can contribute enormously to the diagnosis of sensorineural hearing losses. Plain skull films may aid in the diagnosis of Paget's disease, whereas transorbital views may show asymmetry of the internal auditory meatus in the presence of acoustic neuroma. Hypocycloidal polytomography of the temporal bone will confirm this asymmetry and will also aid in the diagnosis of such congenital abnormalities as Michel's or Mondini's deformity. These x-rays have been used in the diagnosis of cochlear otosclerosis, but some caution must be exercised in making this diagnosis because pathologic sections of a few temporal bones do not correlate perfectly with the roentgenographic diagnosis of otosclerosis. Computerized axial tomograms often help in the diagnosis of acoustic neuromas, other cerebellopontine angle tumors, and other intracranial abnormalities. The resolution of this modality is increasing with each successive generation of scanners.

ELECTROCARDIOGRAPHY

In patients suffereing the Jervell and Lange-Nielsen syndrome, the electrocardiogram shows an abnormally long Q–T interval. These patients often present with syncope and may die from cardiac irregularities, making their diagnosis imperative.

MICROBIOLOGIC EXAMINATION

Microbiologic cultures will identify the organisms involved in the infective causes of sensorineural deafness. Viral studies on serum, stool, and cerebrospinal fluid may be useful in confirming a suspected viral etiology for hearing loss, but the laboratory results are usually not available in time to affect the treatment, and therefore these studies are not recommended.

EXPLORATORY SURGERY

Myringotomy may be used to obtain fluid for culture in patients with serous or suppurative labyrinthitis. A round or oval window fistula may be diagnosed by exploratory tympanotomy. A poststapedectomy granuloma is diagnosed by re-exploring the middle ear. By performing a stapedial footplate tap, perilymph can be collected from an ear without useful hearing, and the presence of acoustic neuroma may be diagnosed by the elevated perilymph protein. In patients with both vertigo and sensorineural hearing loss who undergo a translabyrinthine or middle cranial fossa nerve section, the presence or absence of acoustic neuroma will definitely be confirmed.

VESTIBULAR TESTING

Since the peripheral vestibular system is embryologically and anatomically related to the auditory system, its evaluation in patients with hearing loss is indicated. In the case of acoustic neuroma or other central nervous system lesions, the patient may be ataxic with an abnormal gait. Past pointing and dysdiadochokinesia may be present, and the patient may exhibit instability during the Romberg test. In such cases, with caloric testing, the physician can passively examine the vestibular-ocular reflex with the patient's eyes closed and obtain a permanent record of this examination. It may record spontaneous or positional nystagmus and provide some indication as to whether a problem is peripheral or central in origin. Rotation testing often shows vestibular dysfunction earlier than caloric testing but does not identify the side of the lesion. Stability platforms are being used for postureography by tracking the patient's center of gravity and providing specific information on the status of the vestibular system and central nervous system.

Summary

No one likes to face the realization that their body is not whole or functioning perfectly. Victims of hearing loss have traditionally tried to conceal their misfortune. For far too long, society in general and the health professions in particular have been all too willing partners in this deception. A concerted effort should be made to end this futile approach and replace it with a vigorous diagnostic, therapeutic, and rehabilitative program. An awareness of the underlying pathophysiology and the multiple etiologic factors involved in hearing loss provides a solid foundation upon which to base a thorough evaluation, a diagnosis, and meaningful management.

BIBLIOGRAPHY

Fahy, F. J.: Acoustics. *In* Hinchcliffe, R., and Harrison, D. (eds.): Scientific Foundations of Otolaryngology. Chicago, William Heinemann Medical Book Publication, 1976, pp. 87–101.

Lawrence, M.: Some physiological factors in inner ear deafness. Ann Otol 69:480–496, 1960.

Lawrence, M: Hair cell—tectorial membrane complex. Am J Otolaryngol 2:345–347, 1981.

Marcus, R. E.: Cochlear and neural diseases: classification and oto-audiological correlations. Ann Otol Rhinol Laryngol 83:304–311, 1974.

Meyerhoff, W. L.: Medical management of hearing loss. Laryngoscope 88:960–973, 1978.

Meyerhoff, W. L.: Hypothyroidism and the ear: electrophysiological, morphological, and chemical considerations. Laryngoscope 89:1–25, 1979.

Meyerhoff, W. L., and Paparella, M. M.: Diagnosing the cause of hearing loss. Geriatrics 33:95–99, 1978.

Nadol, J. B., Jr.: Serial section reconstruction of the neural poles of hair cells in the human organs of Corti. II. Outer hair cells. Laryngoscope 93:780–791, 1983.

Saunders, W., and Meyerhoff, W. L.: Physical Exam of the Ear. *In* Paparella, M. M., and Shumrick, D. A. (eds.) Otolaryngology. Philadelphia, W.B. Saunders Co., 1980.

Schuknecht, H. F.: Pathology of the Ear. Cambridge, Mass., Harvard University Press, 1974.

Spoendlin, H.: The innervation of the outer hair cell system. Am J Otol 33:274–278, 1982.

Tempest, W.: Electroacoustics. *In* Hinchcliffe, R., and Harrison, D. (eds.): Scientific Foundations of Otolaryngology. Chicago, William Heinemann Medical Book Publication, 1976, pp. 101–111.

Voldrich, L.: Mechanical properties of basilar membrane. Acta Otolaryngol 86:331–335, 1978.

Zwislocki, J. J.: Middle Ear, cochlea, and Tonndorf. Am J Otolaryngol 2:240–250, 1981.

Peter Hilger
Michael M. Paparella
Robert G. Anderson

2

CONDUCTIVE HEARING LOSS

Conductive hearing loss results from disorders associated with an abnormality in the reception and transmission of sounds through the external auditory canal, tympanic membrane, and middle ear space. Such disorders deserve prompt and thorough evaluation because they may represent a more serious disease, such as malignancy in the nasopharynx, middle ear, or auditory canal. In addition, untreated conductive hearing loss may be the cause of significant and lasting disability, as exemplified by children with congenital conductive hearing loss and consequent language retardation. Finally, even the mildest forms of conductive hearing loss decrease the quality of life by impairing the patient's ability to communicate. Treatment of these disorders is rewarding for both the patient and physician. Conductive hearing loss may present at birth (congenital) or manifest later in life (delayed). Aside from impacted cerumen in the external auditory canal, otitis media is the most common cause of conductive hearing loss and will be discussed in detail in Chapter 3.

Congenital Conductive and Mixed Hearing Loss

Congenital conductive hearing loss can be caused by a variety of disorders, including external auditory canal atresia or stenosis; ossicular deformity, discontinuity, or fixation; congenital cholesteatoma; middle ear effusion; and agenesis of the labyrinthine windows. These abnormalities may occur alone or in association with other regional or distant malformations. Convenient classification systems divide congenital hearing losses into those that occur as an isolated anomaly and those that occur as part of a particular syndrome. Since it is often difficult to determine conclusively whether a defect is genetic, this chapter will indicate hereditary patterns only for those syndromes in which a mode of inheritance has been clearly established.

The signs and symptoms of congenital hearing loss are not uniformly present at birth. However, when a gross malformation, such as aural atresia, is present, the problem is readily apparent. If the child has a more subtle malformation, such as an isolated ossicular anomaly, the hearing loss may remain undetected for several years and be discovered only when the child fails to meet developmental guidelines. It should be noted that up to 30 per cent of patients with congenital malformations of the external or middle ear also have inner ear anomalies. Conductive hearing loss in children is difficult to distinguish from sensorineural or mixed loss because the otologic and audiologic examinations of children are frequently difficult to perform. Fortunately, newer testing techniques, such as impedance audiometry and brainstem response audiometry, are permitting earlier recognition and localization of deficits in the hearing impaired child (see Chapter 8).

Without the "red flag" of a deformed or absent pinna or external auditory canal, recognition of a unilateral congenital hearing loss may be delayed for years. Fortunately, unilateral hearing loss is a less urgent situation than bilateral loss. One normal ear will permit normal speech development, and with few exceptions, children with unilateral conductive hearing loss develop normally from an educational and psychologic standpoint and do not require treatment until later in life when unilateral hearing may become a social or occupational handicap. The patient may then elect to use a hearing aid or undergo surgical correction of the conductive hearing loss.

Sometimes a hearing loss is obvious (e.g., bilateral aural atresia). If it is not obvious, but suspected, owing to a high-risk situation (see Tables 1–2, 1–3, 1–6, and 1–7), the child may be tested by brainstem response audiometry as early as 6 weeks of age. If such testing confirms the presence of bilateral hearing loss, the child should be fitted with a hearing aid or hearing aids immediately. Because the ability to acquire auditory discrimination decreases with age, the child should also begin special auditory training within the first year of life.

When congenital hearing loss is suspected owing to the child's inattention, delayed speech development, or signs of hearing difficulty (e.g., sitting close to the television or personality problems), hearing evaluation and a complete ear examination should be performed as soon as possible. Further testing may then be initiated to define the severity and cause of the hearing loss and to assess other anomalies when present. Appropriate medical and surgical therapy is instituted when necessary, and periodic re-evaluation is performed to rule out progression of the hearing loss. If indicated and if the abnormality is not suitable for immediate surgical correction, the child should be fitted with a hearing aid or hearing aids.

Surgical reconstruction of a bilateral congenital conductive hearing loss should be delayed until the child is 4 to 6 years old. A more accurate audiogram, which will define the conductive or sensorineural components of the hearing loss, can be obtained at that time, and the mastoid air cell system will have increased in size to provide access for surgery. Tomographic x-rays should be obtained to fully evaluate the inner, middle, and external ear. If pneumatization of the mastoid fails to develop, surgery may be delayed indefinitely.

Pinna malformations may accompany defects of the external auditory canal and middle ear, and the appearance of the ear may actually be more distressing to the family than the functional abnormality. Although some otologic surgeons prefer to correct the hearing loss first, the majority will wait until auricular cosmesis and relocation for symmetry have been completed prior to reconstructive middle or external ear surgery. In such cases it is very important to provide the necessary emotional support to the parents. Further, with knowledge of hereditary patterns (see Tables 1–2, 1–3, 1–6, and 1–7), genetic counseling may be offered.

CONGENITAL CONDUCTIVE (AND MIXED) HEARING LOSS WITHOUT OTHER ASSOCIATED ANOMALIES

Canal Stenosis or Atresia

Malformations of the external and middle ear are relatively uncommon, occurring in one of 10 thousand to 20 thousand births. A unilateral anomaly occurs four times more frequently than a bilateral defect and more often affects the right ear. Malformations of the external and middle ear have been found in several studies to be more common in males. Although some investigators believe that the deficit is due to a disturbance in the posterior cranial organization centers, others believe the etiology to be hypoxia from a vascular injury during the development of the branchial arches.

The association between external and middle ear malformations is understandable given their common embryologic origins. The first and second branchial arches give rise to the pinna and ear canal up to the sixth week of embryonic life. Although controversy exists, it appears that the first arch forms the peritragal area, the second arch gives rise to the remainder of the auricle, and the external auditory canal develops from the first branchial cleft. This process is complete by about the 28th week of gestation. Development of the middle ear begins during the third week of gestation, and the ossicles form between the sixth and 28th week. The head of the malleus and the body and short process of the incus are derived from the first branchial arch, whereas the long process of the incus and most of the stapes develop from the second arch. The stapes footplate is derived from the otic capsule. Owing to the common source (first and second branchial arches) and synchronous development (sixth to 28th week), abnormalities of the external ear are often associated with those of the middle ear. In addition, the severity of pinna malformation often provides a crude index to predict the extent of the middle ear abnormality.

A useful classification system considers three grades of ear malformation. The largest

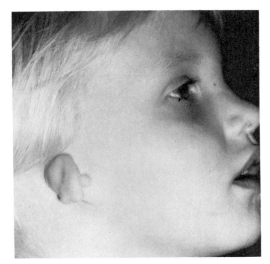

Figure 2–1. Congenital atresia of the external ear.

group consists of minor malformations. The pinna and external ear canal may be normal but often slightly malformed. The tympanic membrane is usually present but thickened, and the ossicles show varying degrees of malformation. The next largest group contains more severe malformations. A vestigial pinna is usually present and accompanied by an atretic external ear canal (Fig. 2–1). The tympanic membrane is frequently replaced by a bony plate, and the middle ear and ossicles again show varied degrees of malformation. The third and smallest group contains the most severe anomalies. The pinna is often absent, and the external auditory canal is atretic. The middle ear, if present, is hypoplastic, and the ossicles are often absent. Unlike the first two groups of malformations, the mastoid air cell system often fails to develop in this group of more severe anomalies, restricting any attempt to reconstruct the ear. As previously noted, sensorineural hearing loss is seen in approximately 30 per cent of ears with external and middle ear anomalies. Those ears with the most severe malformations have the highest incidence of sensorineural hearing loss. The course of the facial nerve through the temporal bone is frequently affected by anomalous development of the ear. Therefore, reconstruction of congenitally malformed ears exposes the facial nerve to greater risk than procedures on normal ears.

A wide spectrum of ossicular anomalies may be seen in congenitally malformed ears. The most frequent include absence of the long process of the incus and agenesis of the stapedius tendon. Other malformations include a deformed and/or fused malleus-incus complex, fusion of the malleus with the external canal atresia plate or epitympanum, partial or total agenesis of the stapes suprastructure (crura and capitulum), bony union of the stapes with the promontory, and fixation of the stapes footplate (Fig. 2–2). Malformations of the labyrinthine windows (round and oval windows) can also be seen in association with various congenital ear anomalies. These defects include agenesis or development in an abnormal position of one or both windows. As previously noted, it is usually impossible to obtain a complete and accurate audiogram until a child is approximately 3 or 4 years old. However, a less precise assessment of hearing is possible early in the neonatal period through the use of brainstem audiometry (ABR) and later through techniques such as conditioned-response audiometry, behavior-response audiometry, and impedance audiometry. If a normal inner ear is present and there is no sensorineural hearing loss, an ear with an atretic external canal, fixed ossicles, ossicular discontinuity, or agenesis of a labyrinthine window will have a 50- to 60-dB conductive hearing loss. Early audiometric testing is important so that the child with a significant bilateral loss can be fitted with a hearing aid or hearing aids.

Roentgenographic evaluation of congenitally malformed ears should include standard mastoid films and temporal bone tomograms. New high-resolution computed to-

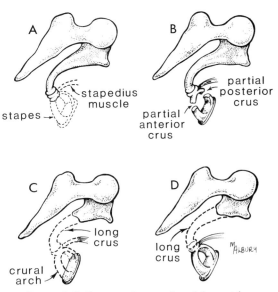

Figure 2–2. Congenital anomalies of the ossicles.

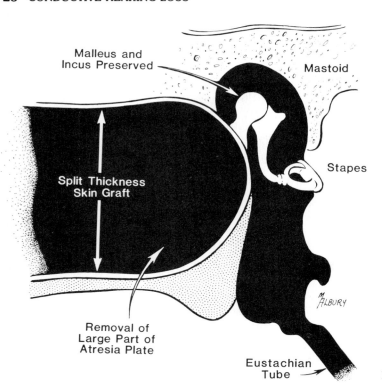

Figure 2–3. Canaloplasty and ossicular reconstruction (type I).

mography may also provide useful information. These radiographs help define the nature and extent of the external and middle ear defects as well as inner ear anomalies, abnormalities in the course of the facial nerve canal, and mastoid pneumatization. They are also useful in the evaluation of congenital cholesteatoma, which can occur with other external and middle ear anomalies.

Surgical reconstruction of the congenitally malformed ear often requires an approach to the middle ear through the mastoid air cell system. The most severely deformed ears rarely have a pneumatized mastoid and often have no ossicle. Therefore, most otologists do not recommend surgery for these cases but prescribe amplification when necessary. Reconstruction of less severely deformed ears is usually delayed until the child is four to six years old, allowing for maximal development of the mastoid air cell system.

There are three principal surgical techniques currently used to improve hearing in congenitally malformed ears. Canaloplasty, tympanoplasty, and fenestration of the horizontal semicircular canal. Mild malformations include those in which the external canal can be enlarged (canaloplasty) and the tympanic membrane and ossicles reconstructed (tympanoplasty) (Fig. 2–3). A thick,

poorly functioning tympanic membrane may be replaced with fascia or skin graft, and involved ossicles may be repositioned or replaced to correct ossicular discontinuity or fixation. The best hearing results are obtained by correcting these types of mild malformations.

More severe malformations in which the external canal is atretic require exposure of the middle ear through the mastoid antrum (Fig. 2–4) and removal of a portion of the bony atresia plate. If a mobile stapes is present with a malformed or absent incudomalleolar complex, a type III tympanoplasty can be performed (Fig. 2–5). In this procedure, a graft, which will function as a new tympanic membrane, is placed in the newly created external canal in direct contact with the stapes. If the stapes is fixed, the surgeon may elect to fenestrate the horizontal semicircular canal. In this procedure, a small amount of bone is removed from the horizontal semicircular canal, exposing the membranous inner ear. A thin graft is then placed over the opening. With this arrangement, sound entering the external auditory canal will displace the inner ear fluids by moving the graft overlying the horizontal canal fenestration.

Surgical correction of moderate ear deformities can improve hearing thresholds to

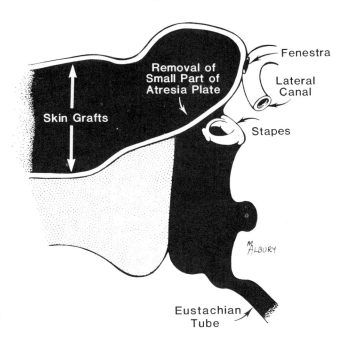

Figure 2–4. Canaloplasty and fenestration of the lateral semicircular canal (type V-A).

30 dB or better in up to 70 per cent of patients. Most otologists recommend delaying correction of unilateral atresia until the temporal bone has fully developed and the patient is of legal age to make his own surgical decision.

Congenital Cholesteatoma

Congenital cholesteatoma is an epidermal tumor, which arises from ectodermal tissue trapped during embryologic development. Although rare, congenital cholesteatomas

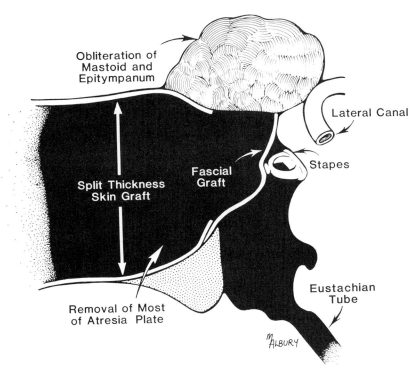

Figure 2–5. Canaloplasty and type III tympanoplasty.

may be seen in several anatomic locations, including the middle ear, external auditory canal, petrous apex, and several sites within the cranium. Intracranial cholesteatomas may cause sensorineural hearing loss but will not be discussed here. Those that occur in the middle ear or external auditory canal can result in conductive hearing loss.

The first branchial groove (cleft) forms the external auditory canal. During the third trimester of gestation, the canal, which is initially represented as a solid core of epithelium, begins to canalize. This process begins at the medial portion of the canal and extends laterally. If the development is arrested before the canal communicates with the external meatus, an epithelialized cyst or congenital cholesteatoma is produced. If the canal atresia is investigated at an early age, the cholesteatoma can be detected and treated before it has produced significant injury. However, if it remains undetected, it will enlarge and may destroy structures in the middle ear, inner ear, mastoid, and cranium.

Middle ear congenital cholesteatoma usually presents as an isolated conductive hearing loss in childhood. No figures are available describing the incidence of this disorder. The conductive hearing loss is due to the mass of the cholesteatoma impeding sound transmission. The tumor may also cause inflammation in the middle ear cleft, leading to middle ear effusion or ossicular erosion. If the cholesteatoma becomes secondarily infected, it will create a tympanic membrane perforation and otorrhea. At this point it becomes difficult to distinguish a congenital cholesteatoma from the acquired type. If left untreated, congenital cholesteatoma will produce signs, symptoms, and complications similar to the acquired type.

Physical examination in the course of congenital cholesteatoma development may reveal a white mass behind an intact tympanic membrane, which may be accompanied by middle ear effusion. X-ray findings are often normal, and the audiologic evaluation will demonstrate a conductive hearing loss of up to 60 dB. Treatment is surgical removal of the mass, and although some conductive hearing loss usually persists, the chances are good that the ear will be trouble-free.

Surgical Considerations. Currently there are two basic approaches to the treatment of aural cholesteatoma. The intact canal wall tympanoplasty-mastoidectomy preserves the anatomy of the external auditory canal by approaching cholesteatoma through both the mastoid air cell system and the ear canal. The open cavity technique, on the other hand, converts the external auditory canal and mastoid into a common cavity. In consideration of the goals of cholesteatoma surgery, the primary objective is to remove all cholesteatoma and thus create a safe ear. Secondary objectives include preservation or restoration of normal anatomic contours and functional capacity (hearing).

The overall hearing results may be slightly better from intact canal wall procedures from open cavity techniques. The major advantage of an intact canal wall is the absence of a mastoid cavity. Patients with open mastoid cavities tend to have a higher incidence of recurrent otorrhea postoperatively (up to 25 per cent), must avoid getting water in the ear, and require cleaning of the cavity on a semiannual or annual basis. The major disadvantage of the intact canal wall procedure is the problem of residual and recurrent cholesteatoma. Since the mastoid is not open for direct inspection, residual cholesteatoma in the mastoid and epitympanum may not be recognized until complications occur. This fact, as well as the known incidence of residual cholesteatoma (15 to 30 per cent), requires that most intact canal procedures for cholesteatoma be performed as two-stage procedures, with the second stage consisting of looking again into the mastoid, epitympanum, and middle ear from 10 to 18 months following the initial surgery. Recurrent cholesteatoma develops from a retraction pocket into the middle ear, epitympanum, or facial recess or from ingrowth of skin secondary to graft failure. It does not often occur in open cavity procedures. It occurs in up to 5 per cent of cases in which intact canal wall procedures were performed. Most surgeons agree that no single surgical procedure should routinely be carried out in every case of cholesteatoma. The two basic approaches are both compromises of an ideal situation that is not attainable surgically; therefore the surgeon must decide for himself which compromise operation he will perform: (1) an open cavity procedure, which has less chance of residual and recurrent cholesteatoma but which requires the avoidance of water and subsequent follow-up and cleaning of the cavity for the remainder of the patient's life or (2) the intact canal wall procedure, which possibly results in better overall hearing and no cavity, but usually requires a second operation to check for and remove residual or recurrent cholesteatoma.

CONGENITAL CONDUCTIVE (AND MIXED) HEARING LOSS ASSOCIATED WITH SYNDROMES

Many syndromes exist in association with conductive hearing loss. This discussion will not be an encyclopedic description of all these disorders but, rather, a brief description of some of the more frequent and important diseases. Although definitive therapy is often lacking, familiarity with these problems and their mode of inheritance aids the physician in providing necessary emotional support and genetic counseling.

Apert's Syndrome

Apert's disease or acrocephalosyndactyly is a member of the group of disorders characterized by craniosynostosis (Fig. 2–6). It occurs once in every 160,000 births, but owing to a high infant mortality rate has a prevalence of 1 to 2 million among the general population. Autosomal dominant transmission is suggested by the few familial cases, a lack of sex predilection, an increased

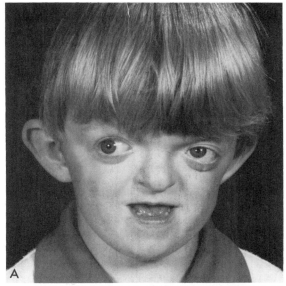

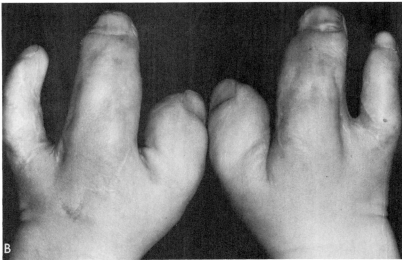

Figure 2–6. *A,* Patient with Apert's syndrome. *B,* Hands of patient shown in *A.* The syndactyly has been partially corrected.

paternal age at conception, and the large number of sporadic cases. Apert's syndrome is characterized by an oxycephalic appearance, hypoplastic maxilla, relative prognathism, pear-shaped nose, hypertelorism, strabismus, and proptosis. Spina bifida has been described in some cases, and many affected individuals have less than average intelligence. Symmetric syndactyly varies in severity from soft tissue fusion to both soft tissue and osseous fusion. The auricles may exhibit a mild microtia or posterior rotation. Described ossicular abnormalities include a fused incus-malleus mass, congenitally fixed footplate, and jugular bulb dehiscence.

Most patients with Apert's syndrome, with or without palatal clefting, have mild to moderate conductive hearing loss with no sensorineural component. Although the hearing loss may be due to congenital fixation of the stapes, the majority of hearing loss in this disorder is consequent to persistent serous otitis media and its untreated sequelae of tympanic membrane perforation, atelectasis, and cholesteatoma. Surgical correction of a congenitally fixed stapes may result in an excessive flow of perilymph through an enlarged cochlear aqueduct.

Crouzon's Syndrome

Crouzon's disease, also known as craniofacial dysotosis, is characterized by cranial synostosis, exophthalmos, hypertelorism, hypoplastic maxilla, relative prognathism, pear-shaped nose, and short upper lip. Premature closure of the cranial structures can cause mental retardation. Choanal atresia and partial anodontia are occasionally seen. It is estimated that about one third of patients with this disease have a hearing loss that is mostly conductive in nature and due to middle ear ossicular anomalies. Crouzon's disease is inherited as an autosomal dominant trait, but many cases occur spontaneously.

Klippel-Feil Syndrome

Maurice Klippel and André Feil first described this syndrome in 1912. It is inherited as an autosomal dominant trait, but affects females more frequently than males. The affected individuals have short stiff necks due to cervical fusion, a low hairline, facial asymmetry, spina bifida, cervical ribs, torticollis, meningocele, cleft palate, and vascular anomalies. The hearing loss is often a mixed type, with the conductive component caused by ossicular abnormalities or fixation and the sensorineural component due to underdevelopment or abnormalities in the body labyrinth.

Marfan's Syndrome

This well-known syndrome is characterized by a tall, thin stature, pigeon breast, scoliosis, lenticular dislocation, joint laxity, high-arched palate, and anomalies of the cardiopulmonary system. It is inherited as an autosomal dominant trait. Deafness is rarely associated with this disorder and, if present, may actually be part of a similar syndrome (keratoconus, myopia, marfanoid habitus, and sensorineural deafness) and not actually Marfan's syndrome.

Osteogenesis Imperfecta

Osteogenesis imperfecta, also known as Van der Hoeve's syndrome, is characterized by a constellation of findings, including frequent fractures following minor trauma, short stature, kyphoscoliosis, blue sclera, and hearing loss. It is inherited as an autosomal dominant trait, with variable expressivity. The disorder is congenital in approximately 10 per cent and "tarda" in the remaining 90 per cent. Complete deafness is rarely observed, but impaired hearing is present in 30 to 90 per cent of patients with the tarda type. Although the hearing loss is generally considered to be a conductive or mixed type, pure sensorineural loss may actually be more common, especially in patients over 30 years of age. The cause of the conductive hearing loss is variable and may occur from obliteration of the footplate by a white, chalky, soft mounded bone (50 per cent); degeneration of the stapes suprastructure and replacement by fibrous tissue (21 per cent); bony closure of the round window (13 per cent); or increased compliance of the middle ear system due perhaps to laxity of the middle ear ligaments and tendons. The basic abnormality appears to be caused by a problem with maturation of collagen fibers and production of thin, loose, poorly formed cortical bone, which has a formation rate of up to three times that of normal bone.

The conductive hearing loss in osteogenesis imperfecta is indistinguishable from that of otosclerosis. Stapedectomy is the treatment of choice in this disorder, resulting in complete correction of the conductive component of the hearing loss in up to 75 per cent of cases. As with otosclerosis, stapedectomy has certain risks, including total loss of hearing in the operated ear in 2 to 4 per cent of osteogenesis imperfecta cases.

Treacher Collins Syndrome

The Treacher Collins syndrome, or mandibulofacial dysostosis, is inherited as an autosomal dominant trait with incomplete penetrance and variable expressivity. Patients with this disorder have normal intelligence. The characteristic facial appearance includes antimongoloid palpebral fissures, lower lid colobomas, malar and mandibular hypoplasia, which produce birdlike facies, and deformed or low-set auricles (Fig. 2–7). Up to 40 per cent of patients have a high-arched or cleft palate, and variable degrees of choanal atresia have been noted. Hearing loss may be sensorineural but is generally conductive in nature. The auricles are deformed in up to 85 per cent of patients, with atresia of the external auditory canals occurring in over a third. The ear canal, when present, is often narrow and tortuous. Surgical exploration of these ears has revealed a variety of findings, including abnormalities of almost all middle ear structures, anomalous course of the facial nerve, absence of the oval and round windows, and obliteration of the connective tissue of the middle ear cavity.

If auditory dysfunction is identified, the use of amplification (hearing aids) must be initiated at the earliest possible age. Consideration for surgical correction of a conductive hearing loss may be entertained when the child is approaching school age. In view of the variety of extreme anomalies that may be encountered, outcome is not always favorable. External canal, tympanic membrane, and ossicular and middle ear abnormalities are reconstructed using standard techniques. Heroic attempts to reconstruct the ossicular chain by drilling out a nonexistant oval or round window may result in total hearing loss in the operated ear, and except in special cases, should be discouraged. When oval and round windows are not defined, hearing aid amplification is the treatment of choice.

Pierre Robin Syndrome

It is uncertain whether the Pierre Robin syndrome is inherited as an autosomal dom-

inant trait with variable penetrance or if it is due to an intrauterine insult during the first trimester of pregnancy. It occurs once in every 30,000 to 50,000 births and is characterized by micrognathia, glossoptosis, and cleft palate. Cardiac defects are present in 15 to 50 per cent of patients, and mental retardation occurs in 20 per cent. A hypoplastic mandible with retrodisplacement of a normal-sized tongue is believed to be the source of the episodic respiratory obstruction in these patients. Defects have also been described involving the eyes and skeletal system. Ear malformations have not been well documented, but those described include low-set ears and cupped auricles. Conductive or mixed hearing loss has also been associated with this syndrome.

Goldenhar's Syndrome

Goldenhar's syndrome or oculoauriculovertebral dysplasia consists of the anomalies of Treacher Collins syndrome (mandibulofacial dysostosis) and hemifacial microsomia and macrostomia. A review of cases in the literature has failed to demonstrate the hereditary pattern. The syndrome is characterized by some or all of the following features: asymmetric skull, frontal bossing, malar and mandibular hypoplasia, nostril hypoplasia, epidermal dermoids, coloboma of the upper lid, anomalies of the vertebral column, including synostosis and hemivertebrae, and mental retardation. Other features include

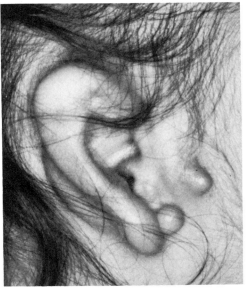

Figure 2–7. Ear deformities in Treacher Collins syndrome.

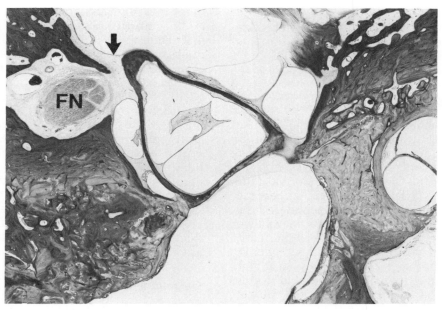

Figure 2–8. Fixation of stapes to the facial nerve (FN) in cretinism. ($\times$ 20.)

microtia, auricular appendages, and first branchial arch fistulas. Various degrees of choanal atresia have also been reported.

Other Syndromes and Conductive (and Mixed) Hearing Loss

Aural atresia has been described in several other syndromes, including trisomy of chromosomes 13, 14, 15, 17, 18, and 21. It has occurred in association with Turner's syndrome. Congenital sensorineural hearing loss may occur in up to 8 per cent of children affected by maternal rubella. Conductive hearing loss due to middle ear anomalies has also been identified in these children. Hearing loss is present in over 90 per cent of patients with endemic cretinism. Conductive hearing loss in this disorder is usually due to middle ear effusion or fixation of the stapes to the facial nerve canal (Fig. 2–8).

Delayed Conductive (and Mixed) Hearing Loss

Most conductive hearing losses are delayed in onset. A functional classification system considers genetic and nongenetic causes (see Tables 1–3 and 1–4). Otosclerosis and Paget's disease are the only thoroughly documented hereditary causes of delayed-onset conductive hearing loss. Trauma, infections, and neoplasm are the usual causes of nongenetic conductive hearing loss. Infectious etiologies will be discussed in Chapter 3.

DELAYED GENETIC CONDUCTIVE (AND MIXED) HEARING LOSS

Otosclerosis

Otosclerosis is the most frequent cause of conductive hearing loss in adult patients with a normal tympanic membrane and no previous history of otologic disease. The diagnosis is likely in a patient 20 to 50 years of age who has a normal-appearing tympanic membrane and complains of a progressive hearing loss (unilateral or bilateral), which, using tuning fork tests, is found to be conductive in nature. A positive family history may be elicited in up to 60 per cent of patients. A conductive or mixed hearing loss will be confirmed on audiogram, and impedance testing (see Chapter 8) will demonstrate normal middle ear pressure, an absent stapedial reflex, and frequently a decreased compliance of the tympanic membrane-ossicular chain. Pathologic evidence of subclinical otosclerosis has been identified in approximately 10 per cent of Caucasians, although it is clinically apparent in only 1 per cent of this race. Blacks and Orientals are affected less frequently. If one parent has clincial otosclerosis, the children have a 20 per cent chance of being afflicted. Some researchers believe that otosclerosis is inherited as an autosomal dominant trait with variable penetrance (25 to 40 per cent), whereas others propose a recessive mode of inheritance. Several studies have shown that females are affected more frequently than males and constitute 60 to 75 per cent of patients with clinical otosclerosis. Studies have also suggested that the hearing loss of otosclerosis may be first noted or exacerbated during pregnancy. The disease has an insidious onset, with two thirds of the cases appearing between the ages of 11 to 30 years. It is usually bilateral (80 per cent) but may develop more rapidly on one side. In addition to developing hearing loss, many patients (60 per cent) complain of tinnitus, and up to 10 per cent have vertigo or dysequilibrium (otosclerotic inner ear syndrome). The vertigo or tinnitus in patients with otosclerosis may be relieved after a successful stapedectomy. Early in the course of the disease, the stapes is not completely fixed and the conductive hearing loss affects the lower frequencies more severely than the higher frequencies. As the disease progresses and the stapes footplate becomes more immobile, the conductive hearing loss may increase to approximately 50 dB.

Controversy exists regarding the existence of sensorineural hearing loss due to otosclerosis. Some otologists believe that otosclerosis can cause pure sensorineural hearing loss. It is proposed that the hearing loss is due to metabolic effects on the inner ear fluids, produced by foci of otosclerosis in the adjacent otic capsule. Others believe that a conductive loss secondary to stapes fixation is always present in sensorineural hearing loss caused by otosclerosis. Despite these differences, there is general agreement among otologists that stapes fixation can cause an increase in bone conduction thresholds, which is most noticeable at 1000 and 2000 cycles per second. This characteristic audiometric appearance (referred to as Carhart's notch), does not indicate a true sensorineural loss. The hearing loss is often improved or eliminated by successful stapedectomy. The sensorineural hearing loss of otosclerosis and its therapy are discussed in Chapter 4.

A review of the histopathology of otosclerosis reveals that the disease is characterized by bone resorption and formation. These activities often proceed simultaneously, and the bone produced is excessively mineralized and acidophilic. The early phase of the disease is dominated by bone resorption and the production of highly cellular and vascular tissue. The later stages of the disease are associated with the production of highly mineralized bone. Several areas of the middle ear may be affected, but the most frequent site is an area just anterior to the oval window, the fissula ante fenestram, which is involved 80 to 90 per cent of the time when the temporal bones have otosclerosis (Fig. 2–9). Extension of the otosclerosis involves the stapedial vestibular articulation, with resultant fixation of the stapes and a conductive hearing loss. Areas less frequently involved include the stapes footplate, the anterior wall of the internal auditory canal, and the round window niche. Invasion of the labyrinthine space rarely occurs.

Evaluation of patients with otosclerosis

Figure 2–9. Otosclerotic focus (O) at the fissula ante fenestram. (× 18.)

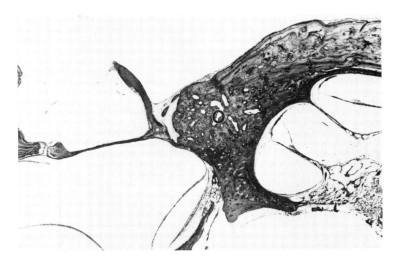

should begin with a thorough otologic history and physical examination, including tuning fork tests. An audiometric evaluation should include air and bone pure tone audiometry, determination of speech reception thresholds, and speech audiometry.

Treatment. Auditory rehabilitation of patients with otosclerosis may be accomplished through surgery or amplification. Surgery may be considered for those patients in whom the anticipated reduction of the conductive hearing loss would eliminate or reduce the need for a hearing aid and for those patients with severe mixed hearing loss in whom reduction of the conductive loss would permit the better use of an aid. The decision regarding surgery should be made only after the surgeon and the patient have thoroughly discussed the potential benefits and risks of both surgery and hearing aid amplification. Surgery should not be considered for those patients with an acute or chronic external otitis or otitis media. Although some otologists believe that a stapedectomy should not be considered in children because of a higher risk of postoperative sensorineural hearing loss and the potential complications of otitis media, children as young as 9 years of age have successfully undergone surgery.

The patient with bilateral otosclerosis who elects to have surgery should have the poorer hearing ear operated on first owing to the ever-present risk of severe postoperative sensorineural hearing loss (1 to 3 per cent). If the first procedure is successful, surgery on the second ear can be considered 6 to 12 months later. The patient with otosclerosis should always be counseled about available options, including using amplification (hearing aid), undergoing surgery, or doing nothing for the present. Since leaving the era when fenestration was performed for surgical treatment of otosclerosis, several procedures have been used on or about the footplate of the stapes. The stapes footplate has been mobilized, fragmented, and removed. It has been partially removed or totally removed with picks, drills, and laser. The open window has been sealed with vein, Gelfoam, fat, fascia, perichondrium, and blood. The gap between the incus and oval window seal has been bridged by a preserved posterior stapes crus, polyethylene tubing, wires, and pistons made of metal and various synthetic plastics.

There are currently three basic methods of "stapedectomy": (1) total stapedectomy, (2) partial stapedectomy (stapedotomy) with footplate preservation (piston technique), and (3) stapedectomy with preservation of the posterior stapes crus. Determination of the advantages of one technique over another must necessarily take into consideration the experience and ability of the reporting surgeon. It is generally accepted that if the footplate is totally removed, the oval window should be covered with tissue and not Gelfoam. If the footplate is preserved and an opening (stapedotomy) is made through the footplate, a piston of various diameters may be placed through the opening, which is best sealed with a small amount of clotting blood or connective tissue. It is suggested by a number of retrospective studies that there is a lower incidence of perilymph fistula and immediate and delayed severe sensorineural hearing loss and less deterioration in bone conduction thresholds in the higher frequencies with the use of the stapedotomy and piston than with the use of total stapedectomy. Preliminary reports also suggest that the use of the argon laser to perform the stapedotomy in the footplate may further reduce the high-frequency sensorineural hearing loss typically seen with total stapedectomy.

Stapes surgery should be performed with the patient under local anesthesia. It usually takes less than 1 hour. Less than a 10-dB conductive loss can be expected in 80 to 90 per cent of patients. Fortunately complications are infrequent, but when they do occur, they can be catastrophic for hearing in the operated ear and for balance. Complications following stapedectomy include acute otitis media (less 1 per cent), bacterial labyrinthitis (rare), meningitis (rare), dizziness or imbalance (about 10 per cent temporary, rarely permanent), sensorineural hearing loss (about 1 to 3 per cent), reparative granuloma (less than 10 per cent), perilymph fistula (less than 1 per cent), persistent or recurrent conductive hearing loss (up to 5 per cent), and facial nerve paralysis (rare). Permanent sensorineural hearing loss, one of the more frequent complications, occurs in 1 to 3 per cent of patients. The etiology of reparative granuloma is uncertain, but the disorder is possibly caused by a reaction to a foreign body or an exaggerated reparative response to surgery, which occurs 1 to 2 weeks following surgery. The major symptoms include sensorineural hearing loss with poor speech discrimination following the initial postoperative hearing improvement, vertigo, and tinnitus. Physical examination may reveal an inflamed drumhead and a negative Rinne tuning fork test. Early intervention is essential and should include exploration of the middle ear and removal of all the granulation tissue, including any extension into the vestibule. The oval window should be recovered, with tissue and the prosthesis replaced. Unfortunately, some of these cases progress to severe sensorineural hearing loss despite therapy.

Oval window perilymph fistula refers to leakage of perilymph through or around the oval window tissue seal. It may occur weeks to years following stapedectomy. The symptoms of perilymph fistula are a sudden decrease and fluctuation in hearing (sensorineural), often with vertigo and unsteadiness, fullness in the affected ear, and occasionally roaring tinnitus. In some patients, the symptoms abate, possibly owing to the closing of the fistula, only to recur as the fistula reopens. The results of the physical examination are often normal, and the diagnosis is made by exploration of the ear. Repair of the fistula with fat or other tissue seal may reverse the symptoms, although the patient often does not recover his hearing.

The chorda tympani nerve is occasionally injured or purposely divided for surgical exposure during stapedectomy. This may cause alternation in taste on the ipsilateral anterior tongue. These symptoms often abate or disappear in several weeks to months.

Paget's Disease

Clinical manifestations of this progressive nonfatal disorder usually begin in the fifth decade of life. Paget's disease is probably much more common than would be expected from clinical diagnosis alone. Autospy studies suggest that it occurs in up to 3 per cent of those over 40 years of age and in up to 10 per cent of those beyond 80 years of age. Most likely it is inherited as an autosomal dominant trait with incomplete penetrance and variable expressivity. Patients rarely present with all the classic signs and symptoms: An enlarged skull, kyphosis, and short stature are rarely seen, and the disorder is often suspected in asymptomatic individuals with the classic lytic lesions seen on x-ray studies. Serum alkaline phosphatase and urinary hydroxyproline are elevated, which confirms the diagnosis. The hearing loss, occurring in up to 40 per cent, may be a mixed type, with the sensorineural

component being slowly progressive and worse for the high frequencies. The conductive loss is usually in the 20- to 30-dB range, with a maximum threshold at 500 cycles per second. The conductive loss may be due to ossicular fixation in the epitympanium or at the oval window. Surgical reconstruction may be considered or the patient can be fitted with a hearing aid. Medical treatment of Paget's disease (calcitonin, disodium etidronate, and mithramycin) does not affect the hearing loss.

DELAYED NONGENETIC CONDUCTIVE (AND MIXED) HEARING LOSS

The following discussion pertains to acquired nongenetic causes of conductive hearing loss. It will consider trauma, neoplasm, and a collection of miscellaneous lesions.

Trauma

Temporal bone trauma covers a broad spectrum of injuries, which range from simple tympanic membrane perforations to complex temporal bone fractures. The most frequent injury is a simple tympanic membrane perforation, which results from rapid compression of air in the external auditory canal. Almost half of these injuries are produced by a slap over the ear and most are located in the anterior and inferior quadrant of the drumhead. The amount of hearing loss will depend upon the size and location of the perforation; small defects may be asymptomatic, whereas larger perforations may produce a 40-dB conductive hearing loss. Altitude changes and diving rarely cause perforations but are more likley to produce middle ear effusion (barotrauma).

Foreign body penetration is another major cause of perforation and may result from the use of cotton-tip applicators, hair pins, or pencils or from inadvertent contact with welding slag. Patients should be warned not to put cotton-tip applicators or other small objects in their ears not only because of potential tympanic membrane perforation but also because of the external otitis that may follow. The traumatic perforation that results from these foreign bodies is often large and located in the posterior one half of the tympanic membrane. Unlike perforations caused by acute pressure changes, ossicular injuries occur in a significant number of foreign body perforations. A useful technique to determine the nature of the hearing loss is to place a small piece of cigarette paper approximately the size of the drumhead over the defect (patch test). If the hearing improves significantly, the hearing loss is probably totally due to the isolated perforation. An ossicular injury should be suspected if the hearing deteriorates or remains unchanged with placement of the paper patch. Eighty to 90 per cent of traumatic tympanic membrane perforation heal spontaneously; however, those associated with water sport accidents may become secondarily infected and fail to heal. The physician should treat patients with this latter type of injury when first seen by cleansing the external auditory canal with suction. Water should not be permitted to enter the affected ear. Antibiotic otic drugs should be reserved only for those ears that actually become infected and start draining. Perforations caused by welding slag rarely heal spontaneously, possibly owing to the cauterizing effect of the injury, which destroys many of the local vessels and retards healing.

Because so many traumatic perforations heal spontaneously, some surgeons recommend no acute treatment. Others recommend elevation of the perforation margins and placement of Gelfoam in the middle ear to support the torn edges. A cigarette paper patch can then be placed over the perforation. If there is evidence of ossicular discontinuity, this may be corrected at a later date, following healing of the perforation, or may be operated on early with simultaneous repair of the torn tympanic membrane. Whenever vertigo or sensorineural hearing loss accompanies the perforation, particularly if it has been caused by a penetrating foreign body, subluxation of the stapes should be suspected. This injury requires immediate surgical exploration to elevate the impacted, medially displaced footplate. When traumatic perforations fail to show definite signs of healing by 3 months, surgical intervention should be considered.

Temporal bone fractures from closed-head injuries are another source of traumatic conductive hearing loss. Seventy-five per cent of patients involved in motor vehicle accidents sustain some type of closed-head injury and up to 15 per cent of these patients have some form of acute otologic injury. Signs and symptoms of the temporal bone fracture depend primarily upon the direction and extent of the fracture. Most fractures run longitudinally or transversely across the axis of the petrous pyramid (Figs. 2–10 and 2–11).

Longitudinal fractures constitute 80 to 90 per cent of temporal bone fractures. They are usually produced by a blow to the temporoparietal area. The fracture extends along the petrous pyramid across the floor of the middle cranial fossa above the middle ear and out the external auditory canal into the squama of the temporal bone. Along its course, the fracture often produces a posterior or superior tympanic membrane perforation and dislocation of the ossicles. Of the three ossicles, the incus is the most frequently affected and may be fractured, subluxated, or severely dislocated into the mastoid antrum or external auditory canal. Less frequently, the stapes suprastructure or the neck of the malleus may be fractured. Sensorineural hearing loss is infrequent, since these fractures rarely extend into the inner ear or internal auditory canal. Facial nerve injury occurs in 10 to 20 per cent of the patients but spontaneously heals in up to two thirds. In over 90 per cent of patients with facial paralysis, the site of injury is in the labyrinthine segment, near the geniculate ganglion.

Patients with longitudinal temporal bone fractures may complain of pain, hearing loss, aural fullness, and tinnitus. True vertigo with nystagmus is infrequently seen and its presence should alert the physician to look for additional injuries to the inner ear or eighth cranial nerve. Cerebrospinal fluid leak and otorrhea may be present; therefore examination of the ear should be performed with sterile equipment. The drumhead can be visualized, and often a perforation can be seen in the posterior superior quadrant. The Rinne test is usually negative owing to an ossicular discontinuity or tympanic membrane perforation. The status of the facial nerve should be assessed as soon as possible, since the time of onset of paralysis may determine the initial mode of treatment.

Transverse fractures usually result from a blow to the occiput and account for 10 to 20 per cent of temporal bone fractures. The fracture originates in the posterior cranial fossa and extends across the petrous pyramid, disrupting the structures in the internal auditory canal and inner ear, and often producing a profound sensorineural hearing loss. The facial nerve is involved in 40 to 50 per cent of these cases, and the injury is almost always a transection of the nerve in

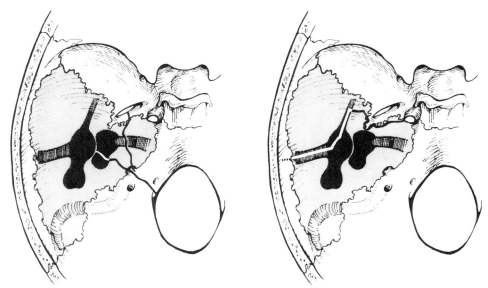

Figure 2–10. Temporal bone fractures.

the labyrinthine segment (90 per cent) or in the internal auditory canal (10 per cent).

Physical examination of patients with transverse temporal bone fractures usually reveals a hemotympanum behind an intact tympanic membrane. This results in a negative Rinne tuning fork test and conductive hearing loss if the inner ear and acoustic nerve have not been injured. Vertigo and nystagmus will be present if the vestibular mechanism has been involved. Not infrequently, the head injury produces a mixed fracture, which displays some of the characteristics of bone transverse and longitudinal fractures.

Temporal bone injury may also cause a sensorineural hearing loss as a result of a cochlear concussion. The loss occurs primarily at 4000 cycles per second and is indistinguishable from the loss induced by noise exposure. Because of the high incidence of hearing loss in patients suffering these injuries, all patients with a closed-head injury should have otologic and audiologic evaluations when clinically feasible. Surgery for conductive hearing loss due to a longitudinal fracture is usually postponed, unless the surgeon wishes to patch the drumhead perforation as previously described. Most patients will not have

Figure 2–11. Temporal bone fracture. ET = eustachian tube; M = malleus; I = incus; C = cochlea; V = vestibule; IAM = internal auditory meatus; EAC = roof of external ear canal; FX = fracture.

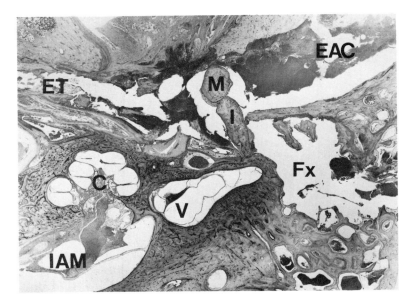

a significant ossicular injury, and the hearing loss will resolve with healing of the perforation and resolution of the hemotympanum. However, if the patient has a persistent conductive hearing loss, ossicular reconstruction is indicated.

Tumors

Tumors of the middle ear are an uncommon source of conductive hearing loss. The discussion of these neoplasms will not be exhaustive but will consider those tumors that occur most frequently. These lesions should always be considered when an unusual clinical picture presents.

Benign lesions include exostoses of the external auditory canal, glomus tumors, papillomas, adenomas, osteomas, chondromas, fibromas, and angiomas. Only exostoses and glomus tumors will be discussed. Exostoses are one of the more common types of lesions and present as smooth bony sessile masses, narrowing the medial portion of the external auditory canal. Some investigators have shown that they arise most frequently in people who sustain repeated and prolonged exposure to cold water. They often occur bilaterally and cause a conductive hearing loss if they become large enough to obstruct the canal or cause squamous debris to accumulate. Treatment consists of surgical removal when the exostoses become symptomatic.

Glomus jugulare and glomus tympanicum tumors, also known as chemodectomas and nonchromaffin paragangliomas, are an interesting group of lesions that presumably arise from chemoreceptor cells located in the adventitia of blood vessels and along various nerves. They occur in several different sites, including the middle ear, neck, and chest. The majority of these lesions are benign, although rare metastases do occur. Since these tumors originate or eventually grow into the middle ear, the usual presentation is pulsating tinnitus due to the extremely vascular nature of the tumor (Fig. 2–12). Conductive hearing loss follows as the tumor enlarges and encroaches upon the ossicles and tympanic membrane. The tumor may continue to enlarge, eroding through the drumhead and presenting as a bleeding polypoid lesion in the external canal. If tumor growth extends through the otic capsule or facial nerve canal, the patient may also have a sensorineural hearing loss or facial paralysis. Extensive tumors can also invade into the base of the skull or into the cranial cavity to involve other cranial nerves.

Examination at an early stage reveals a reddish mass behind the tympanic membrane. Roentgenographic evaluation includes carotid angiography, retrograde jugular venography, and temporal bone tomography. Treatment of these tumors is surgical. Radiation therapy is not curative and should be reserved for palliation only if surgical efforts fail to remove the tumor.

Malignant tumors are the cause of about 1 in 10,000 ear complaints. The auricle is the location of 80 to 85 per cent of these tumors, and the external canal and middle ear each account for about 10 per cent. A malignant lesion should be suspected whenever the patient presents with a friable irregular aural polyp that bleeds easily and is associated with pain (Fig. 2–13). Conductive hearing loss occurs when the tumor obstructs the external auditory canal or invades the middle ear. Evaluation of these lesions should include biopsy, temporal bone tomography, and investigation for distant metastases.

Of malignant tumors, squamous cell carcinoma is the most frequently encountered. It is locally invasive and spreads to regional lymph nodes before producing distant metastases. Facial nerve paralysis associated with this tumor is a poor prognostic sign, indicating extensive spread of the disease. Treatment includes wide local excision or en bloc resection of the temporal bone, combined with radiation therapy. Radical neck dissection may be necessary if regional adenopathy is present. Unfortunately, despite the most aggressive therapy, only 25 per cent of patients with this tumor survive even 5 years.

Rhabdomyosarcoma is the most common middle ear tumor in children. It has a clinical picture similar to squamous cell carcinoma. Triple chemotherapy is currently the recommended treatment, yet the 5-year survival rate is less than 20 per cent. Less common tumors include adenoidcystic carcinoma, basal cell carcinoma, ceruminoma, and various sarcomas.

Histiocytosis-X, although not a true neoplasm, will be discussed with this group of disorders because of its often "malignant" nature and fatal course. Eosinophilic granuloma, Letterer-Siwe disease, and Hand-Schüller-Christian disease are believed to be variations of a single disease process. Eosinophilic granuloma is the most benign of the

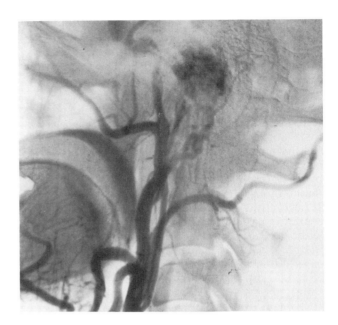

Figure 2–12. Arteriograms showing glomus jugulare tumor.

three and is limited to bone, not infrequently involving the temporal bone. It usually presents in children or young adults as a single or multiple lytic bony lesion. Histologic examination reveals granulation tissue with a cellular infiltrate composed of histiocytes, lymphocytes, eosinophils, and giant cells. Early in the course of eosinophilic granuloma of the temporal bone, the symptoms include otorrhea, otalgia, and a polyp or granulation tissue in the external auditory canal. Later, facial nerve involvement or sensorineural hearing loss may occur. The conductive loss is due to obstruction of the external auditory canal or invasion into the ossicles and middle ear. When the disease is limited to the temporal bone, surgical treatment includes biopsy, surgical curettage, and occasionally mastoidectomy. The most effective current treatment for the limited form of the disease appears to be low-dose radiation therapy. The prognosis for cure following treatment is good. Letterer-Siwe and Hand-Schüller-Christian diseases are more extensive forms of histiocytosis-X that do not regularly involve the temporal bone.

Miscellaneous Lesions Causing Conductive Hearing Loss

Cerumen impaction is probably the most frequent cause of conductive hearing loss. Some individuals produce excessive amounts of cerumen, which can occlude the external auditory canal to produce a conductive hearing loss. Removal can be accomplished with irrigation (warm water using a Water Pik or bulb syringe) or with a cerumen curette under direct visualization. Occasionally the cerumen plug is so tightly impacted that removal is difficult without excessive pain to the patient. This problem can usually be resolved by instructing the patient to use cerumenolytic or hydrogen peroxide drops

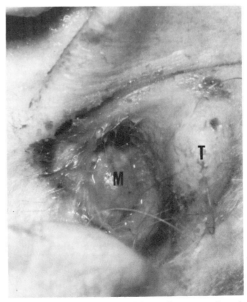

Figure 2–13. Tumor mass (M) in the external auditory canal. T = tragus.

for several days. Removal can then be accomplished in either of the previously mentioned fashions. In extremely difficult cases involving uncooperative children, removal may be accomplished using brief inhalation general anesthesia.

Another disorder that can be confused with excessive cerumen production is keratosis obturans. This is a disease in which the external auditory canal is repeatedly obstructed by accumulation of keratin, squamous epithelium, and debris, which are produced by the drumhead and canal wall. This situation may be coupled with sinusitis and bronchiectasis. It appears that the keratin layer on the drumhead fails to migrate normally across the drumhead and out into the external canal. Regular cleansing is usually adequate treatment, although occasionally canaloplasty with skin grafting of the canal and drumhead is necessary. Inadequate or infrequent cleansing may allow the mass of debris to enlarge and eventually erode through the drumhead and ossicles.

Foreign bodies will be the last source of conductive hearing loss considered. Hearing loss caused by foreign bodies is primarily seen in childhood, although adults may occasionally be afflicted. Rather than hearing loss, the most common complaints are "tinnitus," irritation, or pain. Children may complain of otalgia but are often asymptomatic. If a foreign body has been present in the ear canal for a long period of time, the patient may present with signs and symptoms of external otitis.

Removal of objects lodged in the external auditory canal requires total patient cooperation. If this is not feasible, the physician should consider removal with the patient under general anesthesia. It is important to remember that the first attempt to remove the object is usually the best. Attempts to remove the object in an uncontrolled environment with an uncooperative patient can result in perforation of the drumhead and ossicular disruption. Necessary instruments include a fine suction tip, small alligator forceps, and a blunt hook. Injection of the canal with a solution of lidocaine with adrenalin often decreases both pain and swelling and facilitates removal of the foreign body. The injection should be performed by placing a small bore needle (25- to 27-gauge)

at the lateral end of the external auditory canal. Prophylactic antibiotic otic drops may be used if removal results in canal abrasion.

BIBLIOGRAPHY

Adams, G. L., Boies, L. R., Jr., and Paparella, M. M.: Boies's Fundamentals of Otolaryngology. A Textbook of Ear, Nose, and Throat Diseases. 5th ed. Philadelphia, W.B. Saunders Co., 1978.

Bellucci, R. J.: Congenital aural malformations: diagnosis and treatment. Otolaryngol Clin North Am 14:95–124, 1981.

Bretlau, P., Hansen, H. J., Causse, J., and Causse, J. B.: Otospongiosis: morphologic and microchemical investigation after NaF-treatment. Otolaryngol Head Neck Surg 89:646–650, 1981.

Causse, J. B., Causse, J. R., Weit, R. J., and Yoo, T. J.: Complications of stapedectomies. Am J Otol 4:275–280, 1983.

Gates, G. A., and Meyerhoff, W. L.: Tympanomastoidectomy. In Jaffe, B. F. (ed.): Hearing Loss in Children. Baltimore, University Park Press, 1977, pp. 555–573.

Gorlin, R. J., and Pinborg, J. J.: Syndromes of the Head and Neck. New York, McGraw-Hill Book Co., 1964.

Jahrsdoerfer, R.: Congenital malformations of the ear. Ann Otol Rhinol Laryngol 89:348–352, 1980.

Langman, J.: Medical Embryology. Baltimore, Williams and Wilkins, 1969.

Lawrence, M.: Some physiological factors in inner ear deafness. Ann Otol 69:480–496, 1960.

Marcus, R. E.: Cochlear and neural diseases: Classification and oto-audiologic correlations. Ann Otol Rhinol Laryngol 83:304–311, 1974.

Meyerhoff, W. L.: Symposium on hearing loss—the otolaryngologist's responsibility. Medical management of hearing loss. Laryngoscope 88:960–973, 1978.

Meyerhoff, W. L.: Granulomas and other specific diseases of the ear. In Paparella, M. M., and Shumrick, D. A. (eds.): Otolaryngology. 2nd ed. Philadelphia, W.B. Saunders Co., pp. 1548–1575.

Meyerhoff, W. L., and Paparella, M. M.: Diagnosing the cause of hearing loss. Geriatrics 33:95–99, 1978.

Myerhoff, W. L., and Paparella, M. M.: Management of otosclerosis. In Paparella, M. M., and Shumrick, D. A. (eds.): Otolaryngology. 2nd ed. Philadelphia, W.B. Saunders Co., pp. 1645–1655.

Paparella, M. M., and Meyerhoff, W. L.: Mastoidectomy and tympanoplasty. In Paparella, M. M., and Shumrick, D. A. (eds.): Otolarngology. 2nd ed. Philadelphia, W.B. Saunders Co., pp. 1510–1536.

Paparella, M. M., and Shumrick, D. A. (eds.): Otolaryngology. Philadelphia, W.B. Saunders Co., 1980.

Shea, J. J.: Stapedectomy—a long-term report. Ann Otol Rhinol Laryngol 91:516–520, 1982.

Sheehy, J. L., Gardner, G., Jr., and Hambley, W. M.: Tuning fork tests in modern otology. Arch Otolaryngol 94:132–138, 1971.

Tempest, W.: Electroacoustics. In Hinchcliffe, R., and Harrison, D. (eds.): Scientific Foundations of Otolaryngology. Chicago, William Heinemann Medical Book Publication, 1976, pp. 101–111.

Marcos V. Goycoolea
William L. Meyerhoff

3

OTITIS MEDIA

In its various presentations, otitis media is an extremely common condition, which has major socioeconomic impact. It is clinically important not only because it results in short-term disability (e.g., fever, pain, hearing loss) but also because of its potential complications and long-term sequelae. Early recognition and proper therapy may significantly alter its course and thus reduce these complications and sequelae.

Epidemiology

Because of its incidence and medical and socioeconomic impact, otitis media will be considered separately from other disorders causing conductive hearing loss. Otitis media is an extremely common infectious disease, second in frequency only to upper respiratory tract infections. It is the most common pediatric illness for which antimicrobials are prescribed, affecting 75 to 95 per cent of children by 6 years of age.

Otitis media was a significant cause of infant mortality prior to the discovery of antimicrobials. These drugs have reduced the incidence but not totally eliminated the occurrence of its life-threatening complications. However, with the reduction in frequency of severe complications, more subtle complications of otitis media, such as persistent middle ear effusion with its attendant conductive or sensorineural hearing loss, have become more apparent. These conditions have important sociologic, educational, and psychologic implications.

Definitive epidemiologic studies of otitis media are lacking. Although it is a disease of all ages, otitis media predominates in children. The peak incidence occurs between 6 and 24 months of age and subsequently declines slightly up to age 7 years, at which time the disease becomes much less common. In addition to the age-related incidence, otitis media also tends to occur more frequently during the winter months.

Chronic and severe infections may be more common in males, although there is no definite significant sex predilection. Some racial groups, such as Eskimos and American Indians, have a higher incidence of otitis media; Blacks seem to have less ear disease than Whites. Anatomic and genetic factors definitely play a role in these racial differences; however, the role, if any, played by socioeconomic conditions has not been well defined.

Definition and Classifications

"Otitis media" broadly describes "inflammation of the middle ear cleft" (implying not only the middle ear cavity but also the eustachian tube and mastoid antrum), regardless of the cause or duration of the disease. Otitis media can be divided into acute, subacute, and chronic forms on the basis of clinical signs and symptoms, disease duration, or histopathologic (cellular) changes in the tissues (mucoperiosteum) lining the middle ear cavity.

ACUTE VERSUS CHRONIC OTITIS MEDIA

Histologically, chronic otitis media causes irreversible tissue abnormalities. One sees invasion of the mucoperiosteum by round cells, which are chronic inflammatory cells (lymphocytes, monocytes). Acute otitis media, on the other hand, is characterized by an abundance of polymorphonuclear leukocytes and classic findings of acute inflammation, such as vasodilatation and edema of the subepithelial space (Figs. 3–1 and 3–2). Clinically, the delineation is less easily

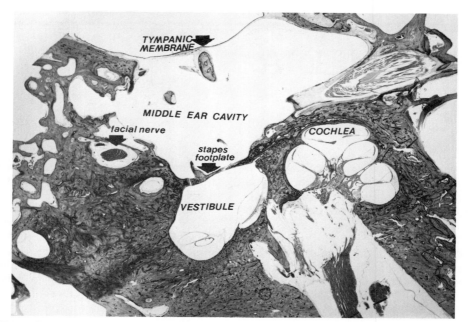

Figure 3–1. Horizontal section of human temporal bones at the level of the stapes footplate. Normal.

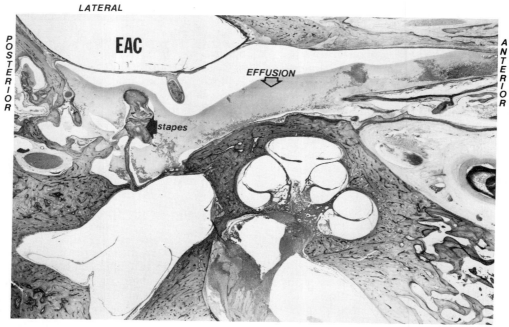

Figure 3–2. Horizontal section of human temporal bones at the level of the stapes footplate, showing middle ear effusion. EAC = external auditory canal.

made. The Ad Hoc Committee on the Definition and Classification of Otitis Media at the Second International Symposium on Recent Advances in Otitis Media with Effusion has arbitrarily classified otitis media as acute when it lasts up to 3 weeks, subacute when it is present for 4 to 12 weeks, and chronic when it persists for 12 or more weeks. By this definition, chronic otitis media can occur with either an intact or perforated tympanic membrane (Figs. 3–3 and 3–4). In the latter case, there may be ear drainage (otorrhea), and in either case, sequelae such as atrophic changes of the mucoperiosteum, tympanosclerosis, ossicular erosion, cholesteatoma, granulation tissue, or cholesterin granuloma may occur (Figs. 3–5 to 3–11). The terms recurrent otitis or otitis prone may also be applied to children who have repeated episodes of inflammation alternating with periods of apparent remission. Acute exacerbation can also occur in an ear with chronic otitis media.

EFFUSION

Fluid in the middle ear cavity is frequently associated with otitis media. There are basically five types of middle ear fluid or effusion: (1) serous (serous otitis media [SOM], (2) mucoid (mucoid otitis media [MOM], secretory otitis media, glue ear), (3) blood, (4) purulent (purulent otitis media [POM], suppurative), and (5) any combination of the preceding, e.g., mucopurulent. It is not yet clear whether these different types of effusions are totally independent of each other (totally different forms of otitis media) or represent different stages of the same disease process. Presently, the clinical differentiation between serous otitis media and mucoid otitis media appears academic, since these conditions occur as a continuum. Since many observers believe that eventually a differentiation between types of effusions will be of etiologic and therapeutic significance, the differences will be described in detail.

Serous Otitis Media and Mucoid Otitis Media

Serous effusion implies a transudate (fluid from subepithelial blood vessels of the middle ear) and contains no cells or bacteria early in its course. This type of effusion is seen in patients following radiotherapy and barotrauma and in those suffering eustachian tube dysfunction. It is important to note that any adult with unilateral serous otitis media should have an examination of the nasopharynx to rule out a coexistent carcinoma interfering with eustachian tube function.

In the pathogenesis of serous otitis media, it is assumed that negative pressure within the middle ear, which occurs as the result of mucosal absorption of middle ear gas during eustachian tube dysfunction, causes transudation of fluid from the blood vessels of the mucoperiosteum. Subsequently, if eustachian tube dysfunction persists, there will be secondary invasion by bacteria. The inflammatory reaction results in proliferation and activation of secretory cells within the middle ear (secretory otitis media). Resulting effusions are a combination of transudation of serum from subepithelial vessels, secretion from goblet cells and glandular structures in the middle ear, and the mucosal absorption of serous fluid already present. As secretory activity persists, the fluid thickens and becomes more viscous. It is then termed mucoid effusion, referring to the mucus secreted by the metaplastic cells and glands lining the middle ear. Clinical experience and experimental evidence strongly support the concept of a continuum from serous to mucoid effusions over the course of time. Unexplained, however, is the finding that, in certain cases, a serous effusion may persist indefinitely or a mucoid effusion may occur without going through the serous stage. Again, the clinical and prognostic differences between serous otitis media and mucoid otitis media are not yet clear, and their recognition is currently of epidemiologic value only.

Bacteriology. Bacterial colonization of chronic serous and mucoid middle ear effusions (present more than 3 weeks) may contribute to the pathogenesis of these conditions. To better understand the pathogenesis of serous otitis media and mucoid otitis media, these middle ear effusions have been analyzed for bacteria by culture and gram stain and for cellularity by Papanicolaou stain. In a study by the author (M. V. G.), effusions obtained at the time of myringotomy and tympanostomy tube insertion from 317 children (509 ears) ages 1 to 11 years were mucoid in 362, serous in 79, and purulent in 60. Mucoid otitis media was found most frequently in younger children, whereas serous otitis media predominated in older children. Bacteria were cultured from 34 per cent of all effusions and in-

Text continued on page 50

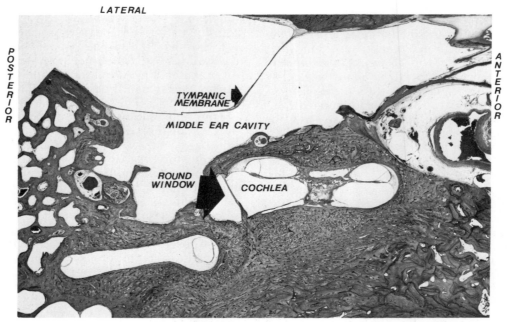

Figure 3–3. Horizontal section of human temporal bones at the level of the round window. Normal.

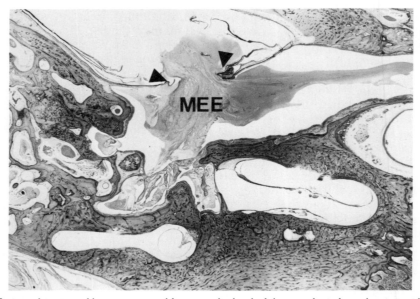

Figure 3–4. Horizontal section of human temporal bones at the level of the round window, showing middle ear effusion *(MEE)* and tympanic membrane perforation.

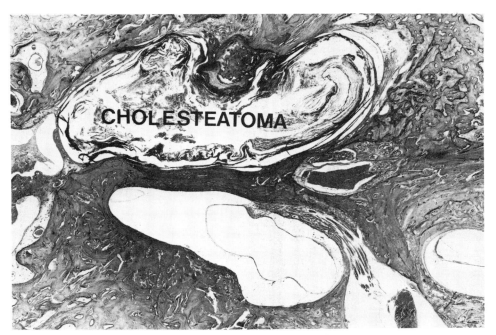

Figure 3–5. Cholesteatoma. (× 10.)

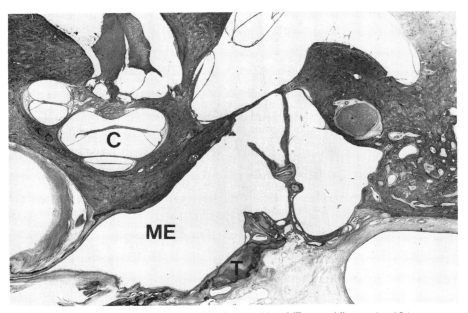

Figure 3–6. Tympanosclerosis (T). C = cochlea; ME = middle ear. (× 10.)

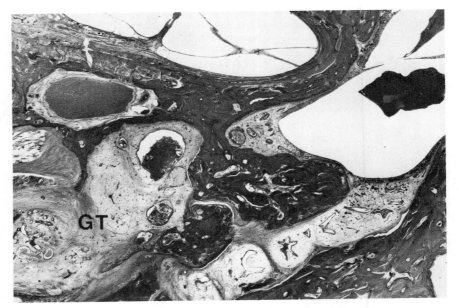

Figure 3–7. Granulation tissue (GT) within middle ear. (× 10.)

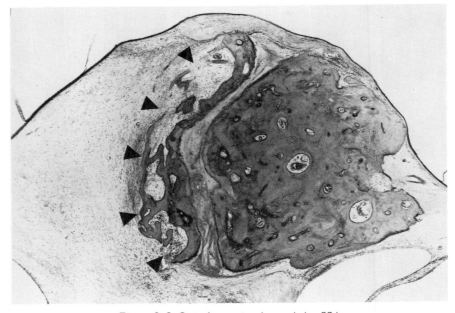

Figure 3–8. Ossicular erosion *(arrows).* (× 32.)

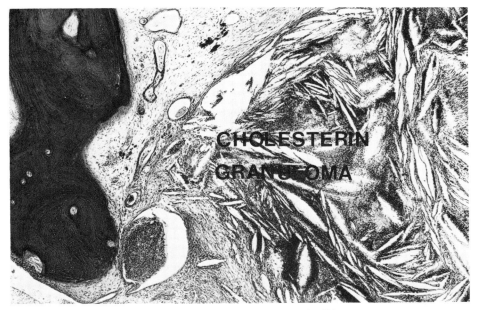

Figure 3–9. Cholesterin granuloma. (× 5.)

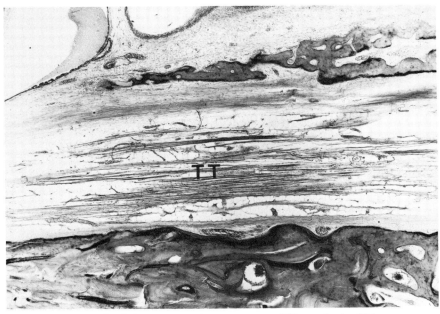

Figure 3–10. Fibrosis around tensor tympani (TT) muscle. (× 32.)

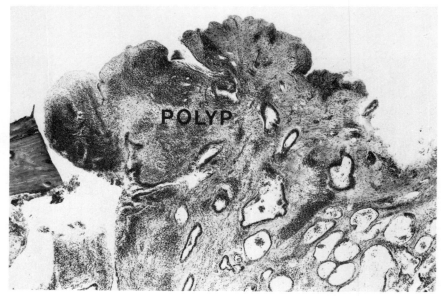

Figure 3–11. Granulation tissue polyp. (× 37.)

cluded *Hemophilus influenzae* (15 per cent), *Staphylococcus epidermidis* (6 per cent), *Neisseria catarrhalis* (6 per cent), *Streptococcus pneumoniae* (4 per cent), and others (3 per cent). An equal percentage of mucoid, serous, and purulent effusions yielded bacteria by culture or gram stain. In sterile effusions, bacteria were observed by gram stain in 16 per cent, and the majority of these organisms were gram-positive cocci. Phagocytes were frequently identified with Papanicolaou's stain on smears from culture-positive middle ear effusions but were less frequent (23 per cent) in sterile effusions. These results suggest that bacteria that are known pathogens in acute purulent otitis media also exist in many chronic serous and mucoid middle ear effusions. The presence of bacteria and phagocytes in these effusions indicate chronic inflammatory stimulation, which may further contribute to the pathogenesis of persistent otitis media with effusion.

Purulent Otitis Media

When a middle ear effusion becomes clinically infected, it is referred to as purulent otitis media. An effusion rich in serum is an excellent medium in which bacteria can multiply. The source of this bacterial contamination is probably the nasopharynx, which communicates with the middle ear through the eustachian tube. Although it is conceivable that some bacteria may be normal inhabitants of the middle ear, there is no definitive evidence currently available that suggests that there is a normal middle ear flora.

Histology. Acute purulent otitis media begins with edema, hyperemia, and hemorrhage in the subepithelial space, followed shortly by local infiltration of polymorphonuclear leukocytes and the accumulation of middle ear effusion if it is not already present. With time, mucosal metaplasia, granulation tissue, monomorphonuclear leukocyte infiltration, and osteitis can be seen.

The exact chronology of these events in the human is not known; however, in the experimental animal with untreated purulent otitis media, hyperemia, edema, polymorphonuclear leukocyte infiltration, and focal hemorrhage in the subepithelial space occur within 3 days of direct middle ear inoculation with *S. pneumoniae*. By 5 days, granulation tissue can be identified, and the epithelium has changed from flat cuboidal to pseudostratified columnar, with goblet cells predominating. Monomorphonuclear leukocytes and osteoneogenesis are present by 2 to 3 weeks.

All these histologic changes have also been identified without clinical changes in the tympanic membrane, suggesting the existence of "silent" otitis media. Other middle ear abnormalities identified in human temporal bone studies are isolated nests of purulent exudate in ears of children with no history or clinical findings of otitis media.

This may provide an explanation for the otitis-prone patient. Also, increased middle ear mesenchyme has been identified in temporal bones from children with coexistent histologic evidence of otitis media, suggesting an association between these two conditions.

Labyrinthitis secondary to purulent otitis media has been described in humans and in experimental animals. The histologic findings range from localized precipitate with occasional leukocytes in the region of the round window membrane to purulent labyrinthitis with diffuse leukocyte infiltration, granulation tissue, osteoneogenesis, and destruction of the membranous labyrinth.

Bacteriology. Bacteriology of middle ear aspirates from children with purulent otitis media has been widely reported. *S. pneumoniae* has been cultured from 25 to 50 per cent of effusions and *H. influenzae* from 15 to 25 per cent. Only a small number of the 83 pneumococcal types account for the majority of middle ear infections with the pneumococcus. *H. influenzae* isolates from middle ears are mostly nontypable, whereas hemophilus isolates in other instances of invasive disease are nearly always type b. The relative incidence of pneumococcal and hemophilus otitis media remains relatively constant between 6 weeks and 13 years of age; hemophilus otitis media does not decrease in frequency after 4 years of age as was true prior to 1960. *Staphylococcus pyogenes* accounted for a significant proportion of effusion isolates 25 years ago; however, this organism is now isolated from less than 6 per cent of effusions. Occasionally *N. catarrhalis*, *Staphylococcus aureus*, and *S. epidermidis* are cultured in pure growth from acute purulent effusions.

Acute purulent otitis media in neonates is often due to coliform bacteria and S. aureus, although common upper respiratory pathogens may also play a role. According to one report, pneumococci and hemophilus were isolated in 67 per cent and coliforms in 23 per cent of effusions from 44 neonates. Coliforms were not isolated from acute effusions in infants older than 6 weeks of age. Several reports emphasize the importance of acute otitis media during the neonatal period and especially in the premature.

Selection of an appropriate antimicrobial regimen in cases of purulent otitis media would be greatly facilitated by direct culture of middle ear effusion. This is difficult and not without danger to the middle ear structures. Consequently, the nasopharynx has been examined as a more accessible source of potential pathogens. Unfortunately, in 50 to 80 per cent of these cases, more than one pathogen is recovered from the nasopharynx, and although in most instances the organism present in the middle ear is also present in the nasopharynx, the multiplicity of potential nasopharyngeal pathogens does not permit upper respiratory cultures to accurately predict the middle ear pathogen.

Nearly one third of effusions from children with purulent otitis media are sterile when cultured by aerobic methods. In one report, anaerobes were isolated in 35 per cent of children with acute otitis media, although organisms were rarely seen on gram stain. Viruses have rarely been isolated (4.4 per cent) from purulent effusions; yet nearly 25 per cent of patients have nasopharyngeal viral colonization, and seroconversion to one or more viruses occurs in 29 per cent of patients. *Mycoplasma pneumoniae* is rarely recovered from middle ear effusions, although mycoplasma seroconversion occurs in 9 per cent of patients. It is not known whether virus or mycoplasma actually enters the middle ear cleft directly, causing inflammation, or if these agents infect the upper respiratory tract, creating suitable conditions for eustachian tube dysfunction and middle ear effusion.

Hemotympanum

Blood in the middle ear (hemotympanum) occurs with barotrauma, in which sudden pressure changes cause rupture of the mucoperiosteal blood vessels. It may also occur in temporal bone fractures with laceration of the middle ear mucosa. The fluid is initially sterile, and the disease self-limiting. Myringotomy is reserved for cases in which resolution does not occur within 10 to 14 days.

CHRONIC OTITIS MEDIA

Histology

Descriptions of the pathology of chronic otitis media (COM) have included granulation tissue, keratoma/cholesteatoma, epidermatization, fibrosis, fibro-osseus sclerosis, tympanosclerosis, and rarefying osteitis of the ossicles, otic capsule, and mastoid bone.

In a review of 123 human temporal bones with chronic otitis media, the senior author identified histologic changes and the order of their frequency of occurrence. The most common finding was osteitis, which occurred in 90.2 per cent of all specimens. Osteitis was followed in frequency by fibrosis of the subepithelial space (76.4 per cent), granulation tissue (69.1 per cent), tympanosclerosis (27.6 per cent), cholesteatoma (14.6 per cent), and cholesterin granuloma (13.0 per cent). Interestingly, tympanic membrane perforation was present in only 19.5 per cent of all temporal bones demonstrating histologic evidence of chronic otitis media. This latter finding conflicts with previous studies that suggest that chronic otitis media is usually associated with tympanic membrane perforation, and it also indicates that tympanic membrane characteristics are not necessarily diagnostic of the middle ear process.

Cholesteatoma is a cystic structure lined by stratified squamous epithelium, resting on a fibrous stroma, and filled with exfoliated keratin. Granulation tissue, which occurs more commonly than cholesteatoma, is a vascularized form of connective tissue associated with an inflammatory reaction. In early granulation tissue, fibroblasts and vascular endothelium predominate. As the granulation tissue matures, it becomes more dense with increased collagen and reticular formation.

Cholesterin granuloma is less frequently encountered than granulation tissue and appears to be a foreign body reaction to the breakdown products of blood (cholesterol crystals) within the middle ear cleft. Cholesterin granuloma can be induced experimentally by injecting blood or sterile suspensions of cholesterol into the bullae of chinchillas with eustachian tube obstruction.

Osseus changes in the middle ear and mastoid can be identified as early as 7 to 10 days following the onset of otitis media and include necrosis, absorption, osteitis, and osteoneogenesis. There are many theories for the observed osseus changes in otitis media, including enzymatic activity, pressure changes, prostaglandin activity, cellular activity, and changes in the partial pressures of gasses.

The exact relationship between tympanosclerosis and otitis media is not fully understood. Tympanosclerosis is usually a sequela of recurrent acute purulent otitis media and appears to be a hyalinization of the submucosal layers of the middle ear cleft. It may progress in severity, causing ossicular fixation or rarely middle ear obliteration. Hypersensitivity has been etiologically implicated in tympanosclerosis.

Histopathologic studies have also revealed inner ear changes in chronic otitis media. In addition to the rare catastrophic occurrence of acute suppurative labyrinthitis, a more subtle labyrinthitis has been identified with chronic otitis media that presumably results in sensorineural hearing loss. The round window membrane appears to be the most common site of communication between the middle and inner ear. Temporal bone specimens demonstrate middle ear inflammation adjacent to the round window membrane, inflammatory changes in the round window itself, and serofibrinous precipitate and inflammatory cells in the perilymph of the scala tympani of the basal turn. Additional findings include abnormal and missing hair cells in the basal turn.

Endolymphatic hydrops associated with otitis media has been identified both clinically and histologically at a frequency of statistical significance. The authors reviewed 560 human temporal bone specimens in which 109 demonstrated the presence of endolymphatic hydrops and 194 evidenced otitis media. Otitis media and hydrops coexisted in 74 cases, demonstrating a statistically significant correlation between the two diagnoses.

Bacteriology

Effusions rarely occur in otitis media associated with irreversible tissue pathology; however, otorrhea is common in this entity. Culture of these often foul-smelling effusions yields Staphylococcus aureus or coliform bacteria, principally Pseudomonas aeruginosa. The role of these microbes in the pathogenesis of chronic otitis media is not understood, although present knowledge suggests that these organisms are secondary invaders of a chronic secretory condition of the middle ear cleft.

Diagnosis

HISTORY

The symptoms of otitis media are often not readily observed in infants and small children. Evidence of acute otitis media or persistent effusion is indirect and has to be sought. The most important source of information is usually the accompanying parent.

A history of allergies, immune deficiencies, bottle feeding in the supine position, and decreased response to sound, etc., should be investigated. A family history of ear and related disorders should also be reviewed.

Infants with purulent otitis media are often restless, unable to sleep comfortably, and roll their heads sideways. There may be periods of crying or pyrexia. If the disease remains untreated, the tympanic membrane may rupture, resulting in purulent discharge and an apparently more comfortable infant. Otitis media may present with diarrhea, which can confuse the diagnosis.

Older children and adults with otitis media exhibit a variety of symptoms, the most common of which is a heavy, plugged-up feeling or a sensation of blockage in the ear. These patients may also have a hearing loss, tinnitus, and autophony. In acute purulent otitis media, pain and fever may be present. Vertigo is occasionally seen but lightheadedness is more common. The patients often have a previous or concomitant upper respiratory tract infection, and if the ear is partially filled with fluid, they may notice improvement in hearing with different head positions. As the otitis media resolves (or in mild cases with eustachian tube dysfunction), a "popping" or "crackling" may be heard in the ears (see Chapter 1 for supplemental information concerning patient histories).

A complete ear, nose, and throat examination is mandatory. Adequate visualization of the tympanic membrane is essential. Occasionally, in the very young, adequate examination is difficult and, for this reason, otitis media remains one of the most frequently misdiagnosed disorders in childhood. Cerumen should be removed from the external auditory canal, as outlined in Chapter 2, and the canal should be examined for evidence of external otitis. Hemorrhagic blebs that result from bullous myringitis should be sought. In otitis media, there is no pain in the canal or tenderness when the examiner pulls the pinna.

Vascularity of the pars tensa, pars flaccida, long process of the malleus, umbo, and the tympanic membrane should be observed. Tympanic membrane retraction, perforation, or tympanosclerosis should be noted. The normal tympanic membrane is translucent, and middle ear structures can occasionally be identified.

An opaque drumhead may replace the normally translucent tympanic membrane. The cone of light has been overstressed as a diagnostic feature of otitis media and may actually be present in otitis media or absent in the normal tympanic membrane. The tympanic membrane, anulus, and malleolar handle may have increased capillary vascularity, which is seen as erythema in these areas. Increased redness and bulging of the tympanic membrane may also occur in a normal crying baby. Sometimes in mucoid otitis media, the malleus handle has a chalky appearance.

The position of the tympanic membrane is difficult to judge unless there is significant retraction or bulging. Tympanic membrane retraction with fluid and apparent shortening of the malleus handle occurs in "adhesive otitis" and in cases with negative middle ear pressure. In adhesive otitis media, the drumhead may also rest upon the incudostapedial joint and can then be clearly seen on otoscopy. When retraction is present, it may be generalized or localized. When it is localized to the pars flaccida, one must suspect primary acquired cholesteatoma.

The location, size, and number of tympanic membrane perforations should be noted. Perforations may be central (not involving the anulus) or marginal (involving the anulus), single or multiple, and located in the pars tensa or pars flaccida. This characterization provides important diagnostic and prognostic information. A central perforation of the pars tensa does not involve the tympanic anulus and is less likely to be associated with cholesteatoma, whereas a marginal perforation does involve the anulus and is more likely to be accompanied by cholesteatoma. The appearance of the middle ear mucoperiosteum may be observed, depending on the size of the perforation. Areas of scarring or tympanosclerosis should be documented.

Middle ear fluid levels or bubbles within the middle ear are occasionally identified, thus confirming the diagnosis of otitis media. If the tympanic membrane is thickened, fluid may not be observed. In such cases, the mobility of the tympanic membrane can be assessed by use of a pneumatic otoscope. By obtaining a tight "seal" of the external auditory canal with the speculum and by applying positive and negative pressure, tympanic membrane mobility can be assessed. In the presence of an intact tympanic membrane, functional patency of the eustachian tube can also be assessed by the Toyn-bee maneuver; anatomic patency can be determined by the Valsalva maneuver and politzerization. These maneuvers are occasionally used therapeutically to help maintain an open eustachian tube in otitis-prone patients.

The Toynbee maneuver is performed by having the patient swallow while the nose is occluded. The eardrum normally retracts inward when a person is swallowing. The Valsalva maneuver, on the other hand, is performed by exhaling forcefully through the nose while occluding it. The eardrum should move outwards with this maneuver. Politzerization is performed by forcing air through one nostril with a Politzer bag while occluding the other. This procedure requires that the nasopharynx be closed. The patient is therefore asked to swallow water or repeat the letter K several times during pressure application. When effective, the patient feels the ear pop. Catheterization of the eustachian tube can also be performed, but it carries with it the risk of traumatizing and subsequently scarring the eustachian tube and is therefore rarely indicated.

Tuning forks should be employed in assessing auditory function. Although available in several frequencies, tuning forks with a vibration frequency of 512 cps are most commonly used. As a minimum, the Weber and Rinne tests should be performed. With the Weber test, maximum sound will be perceived in the ear with the conductive hearing loss, which also will have a negative Rinne test (see Chapter 1).

A nasal examination is also important in the patient with otitis media. The presence of purulent material, mechanical obstruction, rhinitis, or rhinosinusitis can predispose a person to otitis media. Occasionally, correction of a nasal problem is indicated before any middle ear reconstructive procedure is performed, since the surgery may be otherwise unsuccessful in the presence of nasal factors that have a negative influence on middle ear ventilation. Equally important is visual examination and palpation of the soft and hard palate to rule out clefting.

In adults, the oral cavity, hypopharynx, and larynx should also be examined. The nasopharynx should especially be evaluated for the presence of neoplasms in cases of unilateral middle ear effusion (see Chapter 1 for supplemental information regarding the physical examination).

DIAGNOSTIC STUDIES

Diagnostic studies are used to confirm the clinical diagnosis and to answer specific questions regarding the underlying pathophysiology of the middle ear condition. From the audiologic standpoint, air- and bone-conduction pure tone audiometry and impedance testing are usually sufficient for diagnosing otitis media with effusion. The reader is referred to Chapter 8 for the details of these examinations. In the presence of middle ear effusion and an intact tympanic membrane, the audiogram usually shows a mild to moderate conductive hearing loss of 10 to 40 dB. Greater losses should arouse suspicion of ossicular fixation or discontinuity. Tympanometry is very useful in investigating these latter problems. Otitis media can be associated with sensorineural hearing loss, and this loss may be temporary or permanent (inner ear damage). Release of tension on the round window membrane after treatment may account for sensorineural recovery.

Allergy testing and immunologic profiles should be obtained when otitis media is persistent (not responding to treatment or recurring frequently). Although the middle ear is probably not a target organ for allergy (significant levels of reagenic antibody [IgE] are unusual in middle ear effusion), the eustachian tube mucosa is affected in allergic diatheses, resulting in edema of its submucosa and subsequent eustachian tube dysfunction. Allergic diatheses that are responsible for this situation can be the type 1 hypersensitivity reaction due to the release of vasoactive kinins, resulting from the immune complexing of antigens with specific IgE antibodies on the surface of tissue mast cells. It may also occur as the result of cytotoxic antibodies, immune complexes, and delayed hypersensitivity. Total IgE levels can be measured in the serum as well as in the middle ear effusion itself. In addition, the radioallergosorbent test (RAST) can be used for specific antigens or skin testing may be employed. The application and explanation of most of these allergic evaluations is beyond the scope of this work.

Infrequently, roentgenographic studies may be helpful in evaluating the patient with otitis media. Mastoid x-rays are not routinely obtained except when the case is long-standing, when complications are suspected, or when x-rays are required preoperatively.

The middle ear normally communicates with the mastoid air cell system, and in most cases of acute otitis media, the mastoid air cell system appears hazy. This radiographic finding may result in the incorrect diagnosis of acute mastoiditis.

In persistent cases of otitis media, lateral soft tissue x-rays with special views of the nasopharynx are useful to assess the presence of masses (adenoids or tumors) occupying the nasopharyngeal space. Paranasal sinus x-rays are also of value in ruling out concomitant sinusitis, which could require therapy. As many as 40 per cent of children with middle ear effusion will have associated maxillary sinusitis, and over 75 per cent of these middle ear effusions will clear with irrigation of the involved sinuses.

Cultures of middle ear effusions are not routinely obtained unless recurrent episodes of otitis media occur in spite of adequate treatment, a complication of otitis media is imminent, a mucociliary or immunologic disorder is present, or the case is resistant to the usual treatment. Cultures should be obtained while performing the myringotomy, since fluid allowed to contact the external auditory canal after myringotomy becomes contaminated.

Etiology

There are many predisposing factors to otitis media, some of which are mutually inclusive and others of which are not very clear or well defined. These factors include eustachian tube dysfunction, local or regional infection (viral, bacterial, fungal), barotrauma, alterations in the host immune system, disturbance of mucociliary clearance, regional deformities (e.g., nasal septal deviation and choanal atresia), allergy, environmental toxins, socioeconomic factors, and race.

It is generally believed that adequate function of the eustachian tube is of paramount importance for a healthy middle ear. In fact, eustachian tube dysfunction may be the primary mechanism through which many disorders affect the middle ear (e.g., regional infection, mucociliary disorders, allergy). There is abundant clinical and experimental evidence supporting this fact. Animals with experimentally obstructed eustachian tubes consistently develop otitis media, with histopathologic changes in the mucoperiosteum that mimic the changes seen in human temporal bones from patients with otitis media. Eustachian tube dysfunction may be the result of neuromuscular abnormalities (e.g., cleft palate and paralysis of the fifth cranial nerve), mechanical obstruction (e.g., adenoid hypertrophy, nasopharyngeal tumor, scar formation), subepithelial edema (e.g., allergy, regional infection, or neoplasm), or disturbance of mucociliary clearance.

Function of the tensor veli palatini muscle is essential for function of the eustachian tube. Otitis media is almost universal in individuals with cleft palate owing to functional failure of the tensor veli palatini muscle, which normally inserts in the midline of the palate. Similarly, patients suffering denervation of the tensor veli palatini muscle, which occasionally happens following surgery on the gasserian ganglion for tic douloureux, develop ipsilateral middle ear effusion. Experimental animals that undergo sagittal clefting of the soft palate develop middle ear effusion within 24 hours, and the histology of the epithelium and subepithelial space closely resembles that of humans with cleft palate and middle ear effusion.

Direct mechanical obstruction of the eustachian tube may result from nasopharyngeal neoplasm (carcinoma in adults, nasopharyngeal angiofibroma in young boys); from scarring of the eustachian tube orifice, which occasionally follows vigorous adenoidectomy; or from adenoid hypertrophy itself. Mechanical obstruction of the eustachian tube does not allow for equalization of middle ear pressure and therefore results in negative middle ear pressure and subsequent effusion. Thirty per cent of nasopharyngeal tumors in adults present as otitis media, and it is therefore important to examine the nasopharynx in anyone with otherwise unexplained otitis media, especially the adult patient with unilateral middle ear effusion. Adenoid hypertrophy has long been considered to be an etiologic factor in the development of otitis media. Although the exact role of adenoid hypertrophy in otitis media is not well defined and is currently under investigation, the surgical removal of this structure has been and continues to be a common procedure in children with otitis media. Chronologically, the period of maximum adenoid hyperplasia corresponds to the peak age incidence of otitis media, lending support to a cause-and-effect relationship.

There are several known mechanisms that result in subepithelial edema and narrowing of the eustachian tube lumen. Eventually these factors can lead to eustachian tube dysfunction, negative middle ear pressure, and middle ear effusion. Allergic diatheses, in which the upper respiratory tract is the target organ, result in degranulation of the subepithelial mast cells and release of vasoactive kinins. The fluid that escapes from the vessels of the subepithelial space results in subepithelial edema. Blockage or stasis of the regional lymphatics may also result in subepithelial edema of the eustachian tube. In addition to allergies, infections or neoplasms in the regions that share the lymphatic drainage of the eustachian tube (e.g., maxillary sinus carcinoma or infection, adenoiditis, nasopharyngitis, or nasopharyngeal or hypopharyngeal cancer) may also result in middle ear effusion.

Disturbances of mucociliary clearance may cause eustachian tube dysfunction and otitis media. Both hereditary and acquired disorders can affect the eustachian tube and middle ear by this mechanism. The immotile cilia syndrome and Kartagener's syndrome are two congenital conditions that result in decreased mucociliary clearance and an increased incidence of otitis media. Because of abnormal mucociliary clearance, children with these disorders have multiple episodes of upper respiratory tract infections throughout childhood, requiring repeated treatment with antimicrobials. For this reason they present an otologic problem owing to the frequency of middle ear disease. Because of the unusual middle ear pathogens, a diagnostic myringotomy and culture may be indicated before starting antimicrobial therapy for an episode of acute purulent otitis media. Children with cystic fibrosis also have a mucociliary clearance problem, resulting in frequent upper respiratory tract infections. Unlike the children with Kartagener's syndrome and the immotile cilia syndrome, children with cystic fibrosis do not seem to have an increased incidence of otitis media. Again, because they are exposed to many antimicrobials, they also should have a diagnostic myringotomy and a culture made of middle ear effusion before treatment for acute purulent otitis media begins.

Environmental factors (e.g., fumes, cigarette smoke, radiation therapy) may result in altered mucociliary clearance and an increased incidence of middle ear disease. Irritation from fumes and cigarette smoke results in decreased surface active substance of the eustachian tube and causes a metaplastic change in the epithelium of the nasopharynx and eustachian tube orifice from its normal respiratory type to stratified squamous epithelium. With repeated insults, this condition can become refractory to treatment. It is also important to note that a badly deviated nasal septum, because of its effect on normal nasal and nasopharyngeal airflow, may have a similar effect on eustachian tube function.

Viral upper respiratory tract infections, particularly those of the nasopharynx and paranasal sinuses, frequently result in otitis media. Although the exact pathophysiology of this association is not completely understood, animal experiments demonstrate direct involvement of the eustachian tube epithelial cells by the viral agents, with perinuclear inclusion bodies and loss of cilia. Ineffective mucociliary clearance ensues, resulting in decreased eustachian tube function, negative middle ear pressure, and middle ear effusion. Concomitant with these local and regional events is a systemic decrease in polymorphonuclear leukocyte chemotactic activity and chemiluminescence. Some investigators suggest that the combination of these events predisposes the child with viral upper respiratory tract infection to recurrent otitis media. Extensive experimental work in animals supports this theory.

Occasionally sudden changes in barometric pressure cause a sudden change in middle ear pressure relative to the environment, with consequent transudate or hemorrhage into the middle ear. This occurs primarily as result of flying and scuba diving, but probably does not occur without one of the previously mentioned factors that affects eustachian tube function.

In a way, socioeconomic factors also seem to play a role in the development of otitis media. Although wealth itself does not influence the condition, lifestyle may. The infant that is left in a day care center is going to have significantly greater exposure to viral and bacterial pathogens than the infant that stays at home. Similarly, the infant that is fed in the supine position with a propped up bottle is more susceptible to otitis media than one that is held upright while being fed.

Racial characteristics seem to play a role

in the incidence of otitis media. This disorder appears to be more common in the Eskimo and Indian populations of the Americas than in individuals of European extract. Blacks, on the other hand, seem to have a lower incidence of middle ear disease than Whites.

Questions still remain about the pathogenesis of otitis media. Patients may have one or two episodes only, and in some patients, the otitis media episodes persist, becoming a lifetime problem.

Certainly many of the factors previously mentioned contribute to the chronicity of some cases. Although eustachian tube dysfunction appears to be the most important factor, in the last few years a number of immunologic studies have indicated that immunologic deficiencies or temporary immaturity of the immune system plays a decisive role in the pathogenesis of childhood otitis media.

In addition, there are a number of ill-defined factors in the pathogenesis of otitis media that seem to be important, such as environment, general health and vigor, anatomic variabilities, racial characteristics, and familial trends. Finally, inadequate or premature antimicrobial therapy has been considered by some authors to be an important cause of persistent low-grade infections, recurrent acute infections, or chronic otitis media.

Complications and Sequelae

COMPLICATIONS

Life-threatening complications of otitis media are always a possibility because of the proximity of the central nervous system to the middle ear. In the pre-antibiotic era, Politzer stated that "the temporal bone has four sides; the outside is bounded by life, from which there comes the opening of the auditory canal, one form of our appreciation of what life means; on the other three sides this bone is bounded by death." Fortunately, with the advent of antimicrobials and increasing awareness on the part of physicians and the public regarding the potential seriousness of this disease, earlier identification and treatment have reduced the incidence the lethal complications. Unfortunately, however, complications still exist, and in some cases, not even the best treatment available will prevent sequelae. Important

factors in the development of complications include the infecting agent, the adequacy of treatment, and the resistance of the infected individual.

Spread of infection from the middle ear to adjacent structures can occur by three basic pathways: (1) extension through preformed pathways, such as the round window (Fig. 3–12); congenital bony dehiscences, or dehiscences resulting from fractures or surgery; (2) extension by bone erosion secondary to inflammatory processes, such as a cholesteatoma and granulation tissue; and (3) extension by thrombophlebitis through the venous channels near the infected site, such as the lateral sinus.

Facial Paralysis

Facial paralysis may occur in acute otitis media secondary to the spread of infection through a dehiscence of the bony facial canal, which is present in over 50 per cent of all ears. Myringotomy for drainage of purulent effusion and antibiotics effect a cure in the great majority of cases. Decompression of the facial nerve is reserved for those cases in which despite proper initial therapy, the nerve undergoes axonal degeneration, as diagnosed by electrical testing. On the other hand, facial paralysis occurring as a result of chronic otitis media indicates a serious complication, which demands prompt surgical decompression of the nerve. Facial nerve paralysis in this condition implies erosion of the bony canal by a chronic inflammatory process, with direct involvement of the nerve. In these cases, the nerve sheath (epineurium) should probably not be opened because the ingrowth of fibrous tissue could potentially decrease the overall recovery.

Labyrinthitis

Inflammation of the inner ear may occur secondary to otitis media and can be serous or suppurative (purulent) in nature (Fig. 3–13). Symptoms of labyrinthitis include sensorineural hearing loss, tinnitus, and vertigo, and any patient with otitis media who develops these symptoms should be suspected of having labyrinthitis. Serous labyrinthitis is histologically characterized by a serous precipitate in the labyrinth, whereas purulent labyrinthitis is marked by numerous inflammatory cells. Serous labyrinthitis is

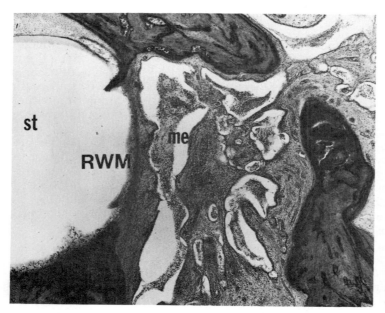

Figure 3–12. RWM = round window membrane; me = middle ear; st = scala tympani. (× 35.)

probably a form of sterile inflammation secondary to exposure to toxic materials which cross the round window membrane or oval window anulus. It is usually a self-limiting disorder, with reversible damage. Purulent labyrinthitis, on the other hand, occurs as the result of direct spread of infection from the middle ear, retrograde invasion of infection through the internal auditory canal or cochlear aqueduct in patients with menin-

gitis, or transmission of infection by way of vascular channels in patients with septicemia. Suppurative labyrinthitis usually results in total loss of hearing and equilibrium due to destruction of inner ear membranes. In cases of severe suppurative labyrinthitis, osteoneogenesis may totally replace the normal anatomic structures of the inner ear (Fig. 3–14). Frequently, it is impossible to differentiate serous from suppurative labyrinthitis

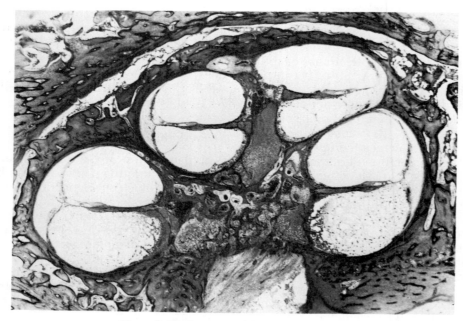

Figure 3–13. Suppurative labyrinthitis. (× 24.)

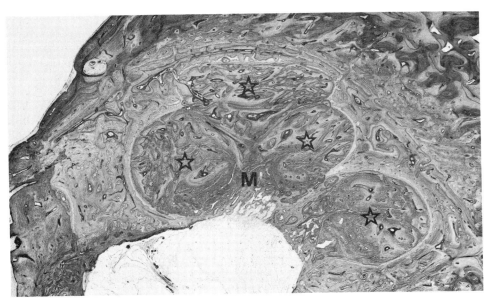

Figure 3–14. Labyrinthitis ossificans (stars); modiolus (M). ($\times$ 20.)

until the episode has resolved. Preservation of hearing and vestibular function would suggest a serous labyrinthitis. Because of this difficulty in distinguishing between the two types, any suspected case should be treated as suppurative labyrinthitis. The treatment is hospitalization, hydration (vomiting often occurs), antimicrobials, antivertiginous medications (e.g., diazepam), and myringotomy. When the patient is stable, further surgical intervention may be considered if the inner ear infection is caused by chronic otitis media.

In addition to serous and suppurative labyrinthitis, a third type of labyrinthitis, localized labyrinthitis or perilabyrinthitis, may occur. This is due to erosion (fistula) of the cochlea or, more commonly, one of the semicircular canals by an inflammatory process, such as cholesteatoma. Like other forms of labyrinthitis, this disorder may result in vertigo and sensorineural hearing loss. In addition to the hearing loss, patients with localized labyrithitis may have a positive fistula test (nystagmus when pressure is applied to the external auditory canal).

Coalescent Mastoiditis

If, despite therapy, acute purulent otitis media does not resolve within the expected period of time, pus that has accumulated under pressure may lead to erosion of the fine bony partitions of the mastoid cavity (coalescent mastoiditis). This condition should be suspected in any patient who has had acute purulent otitis media for about 2 weeks or longer, with or without an aural discharge, and who develops recurrence of pain, fever, and mastoid tenderness. A subperiosteal abscess can also occur and may present as a postauricular abscess (swelling behind the ear with displacement of the auricle forward, outward, and downward), zygomatic abscess (swelling in front and above the ear), and Bezold's abscess (abscess formed by perforation of the tip of the mastoid, with extension down to the posterior triangle of the neck). The diagnosis is confirmed by mastoid x-rays, which demonstrate opacification of the air cells and a decrease in the fine bony septations. The treatment of choice is mastoidectomy and antimicrobial therapy.

Petrositis

Petrositis is the spread of inflammation to the air cells of the petrous apex of the temporal bone. This complication of otitis media occurs between 10 and 50 days following the onset of acute purulent otitis media. Owing to its anatomic relationship to cranial nerves V and VI, this disease may result clinically in paralysis of the lateral rectus muscle and pain in the distribution of the fifth cranial nerve. These two findings plus otitis media have been termed Gradenigo's syndrome. The suspected diagnosis can be confirmed by mastoid x-rays. The treatment of choice includes intensive antimicrobial therapy and surgical intervention, consisting of petrous apicectomy.

Meningitis

Meningitis is the most common intracranial complication of acute purulent otitis media. Any patient with unexplained meningitis should be carefully evaluated for otitis media. Inflammation of the meninges can occur by direct extension of infection from the middle ear or by direct extension due to bony erosion. When dealing with meningitis secondary to acute purulent otitis media, the treatment is medical unless there are recurrent episodes of the meningitis. With recurrent meningitis, exploration of the middle ear and mastoid is indicated in an effort to identify the pathway of communication. The organisms involved are usually S. pneumoniae, H. influenzae, or S. pyogenes. When meningitis occurs as the result of chronic otitis media, surgical intervention is required in addition to antimicrobial therapy for the microorganisms, which are usually gram-negative rods.

Lateral Sinus Thrombophlebitis

Lateral sinus thrombophlebitis develops as a consequence of erosion in the bony covering of the lateral sinus (behind the mastoid). In this disorder, an initial perisinus abscess forms, which is followed by the development of a thrombus within the sinus itself. This complication should be suspected in any patient with otitis media who develops persistent unexplained fever of the septic or "picket-fence" variety. There may be associated progressive anemia, emaciation, and obstruction of venous return from the head (causing headaches). Blood cultures may be positive. Venography will confirm the diagnosis. Treatment is antimicrobial therapy, surgical ligation of the internal jugular vein, and mastoidectomy. Occasionally, thrombophlebitis of the lateral sinus may cause thrombophlebitis of the mastoid emissary vein. The postauricular edema that results from thrombosis of this vein is called Greisinger's sign.

Otitic Hydrocephalus

Otitic hydrocephalus is a complication of otitis media. It is characterized by increased cerebrospinal fluid pressure, caused by fail-

ure of the arachnoid granulations to absorb the fluid or by dural sinus thromboses following meningeal infection and inflammation from the middle ear. This complication should be suspected in patients who develop headache, sixth nerve paralysis, and papilledema following several weeks of purulent otitis media. The diagnosis is confirmed by lumbar puncture. Treatment is reduction of intracranial pressure with repeated lumbar punctures, systemic steroids, and/or shunting procedures. The pressure usually returns to normal after several weeks to months. The treating physician should be aware of the possibility of herniating the cerebral peduncles through the foramen magnum if repeated lumbar punctures are considered.

Intracranial Abscesses

Intracranial abscesses caused by otitis media may occur at different sites. These locations may be extradural (outside dura matter), subdural (between dura matter and arachnoids), intracerebral, or intracerebellar. Although temporal headaches and occasional temporal lobe seizures may suggest the diagnosis, the signs and symptoms may be nonspecific. Nausea and vomiting are frequent symptoms. Diagnosis is confirmed by brain scan.

Other Complications

Further complications of otitis media include sensorineural hearing loss and endolymphatic hydrops. Because definite experimental evidence for the pathogenesis is lacking, the etiology of these problems is currently under investigation. It seems that in certain forms of otitis media, toxins or enzymes reach the inner ear through the round window membrane and cause these pathologic changes.

SEQUELAE

For practical purposes, complications and sequelae are mentioned separately. It should be understood, however, that they can occur in such a way that it is difficult to define what is a complication and what is a sequela. It is also important to keep in mind that otitis media implies not only involvement of the middle ear space itself but also its contents and walls (e.g., mucoperiosteum, ossicles, muscles, tympanic membrane). Some or all these structures may be involved. In some cases, otitis media leads to a continuum of changes that result in sequelae such as tympanosclerosis and ossicular erosion (see Fig. 3–6 and 3–8).

As a result of otitis media, the tympanic membrane may become atrophic owing to loss or atrophy of the middle layers (lamina propria and fibrous layers), leaving only the epithelial layers. This results in a thin, weak, transparent membrane, which is frequently seen in chronic otitis but is usually of little clinical significance. If the atelectatic area constitutes a small region of the tympanic membrane, no treatment is necessary. On the other hand, atelectasis of the entire drumhead may lead to recurrent otorrhea, conductive hearing loss, and cholesteatoma and requires a tympanoplasty to replace or reinforce the atelectatic drumhead. Persistent perforations of the tympanic membrane require surgical repair. The middle ear muscles (tensor tympani and stapedius) are also involved in the general process of otitis media and may become fibrosed, stiffening the ossicular chain and interfering with sound conduction (see Fig. 3–10). These muscles may be lysed at the time of middle ear surgery to alleviate this problem.

Inflammatory processes of the middle ear are also capable of causing ossicular destruction. The degree of erosion will depend on the nature and extent of the process. The most common site of erosion is the long process of the incus, although total erosion of all the ossicles may occur, leaving only the stapes footplate. Conductive hearing loss is the consequence of this occicular chain discontinuity and can be treated surgically. The diagnosis should be suspected in anyone with a conductive hearing loss and a history of otitis media, whether the tympanic membrane appears normal or diseased. In the case of an intact tympanic membrane, the diagnosis of ossicular discontinuity can be confirmed by identifying tympanic membrane hypermobility by impedance audiometry (see Chapter 8).

Tympanosclerosis (hyalinized collagen in the lamina propria) may occur anywhere in the mucoperiosteum of the middle ear cleft. It may involve the stapes, causing secondary fixation and conductive hearing loss. It has been reported that this condition may be observed in up to 7.5 per cent of patients with tympanomastoidectomies. Tympanosclerotic areas frequently occur in the tympanic membrane (e.g., myringosclerosis), typically in the pars tensa. There is little

clinical significance to this latter finding. Although several theories have been presented to explain the etiology of tympanosclerosis, the cause remains unknown.

Granulation tissue may occur in the mucoperiosteum and is frequently quite active, causing a significant degree of bone erosion (see Fig. 3–8). It may be associated with many complications, such as abscesses and thrombophlebitis. Granulation tissue may be viewed through a tympanic membrane perforation or identified at surgery. It may also present as blood otorrhea and is part of the generalized picture of active chronic otitis media with otorrhea. Granulation tissue is removed in the course of tympanomastoid surgery for chronic otitis media. Ear drops may reduce the severity of the problem but rarely result in a cure.

Cholesteatoma, like granulation tissue, can also result in bone erosion and destruction, with similar complications. Cholesteatoma is misplaced stratified keratinizing squamous epithelium, which tends to enlarge with time. Enzymatic and mechanical pressure capabilities cause the many complications of cholesteatoma (see Fig. 3–5).

There are three basic forms of cholesteatoma and several different nondefinitive theories about their origin and pathogenesis. Regardless of the origin and pathogenesis, cholesteatomas may present at almost any age. Treatment for all three forms is surgical, and the extent of the operation depends on the extent of the disease.

The first type of cholesteatoma, congenital cholesteatoma, is the least common variety and is believed to result from embryologically trapped squamous epithelium. Known also as epidermoid inclusion cysts, congenital cholesteatomas may occur in any bone. Symptoms begin insidiously and depend on the location. When arising from the petrous apex, the presentation may be identical to that of an acoustic neuroma. When it arises in the middle ear cleft, a conductive hearing loss is the main symptom. The tympanic membrane remains intact until late in the disease, when coexistant infection and growth result in tympanic membrane rupture.

The second and third types of cholesteatoma are primary acquired and secondary acquired cholesteatoma. Primary acquired cholesteatoma begins as a retraction pocket in the pars flaccida. Uninterrupted, this process will progress through Prussak's space, the area between the pars flaccida and neck of the malleus (see Chapter 1), and into the attic, antrum, and mastoid. Otorrhea and conductive hearing loss become apparent in this otherwise silent process when contamination from the external auditory canal results in associated infection. Secondary acquired cholesteatoma occurs following a tympanic membrane perforation. As the epithelium migrates into the middle ear, it tends to follow the path of least resistance, sometimes resulting in the formation of a "pearl." Destruction of adjacent structures is the result of pressure, infection, and enzyme activity.

Cholesterin granuloma, another sequela of otitis media, is a reactive foreign body response of the mucoperiosteum to the presence of cholesterol crystals (a breakdown product of blood). Histologically, it is characterized by cholesterol crystals surrounded by inflammatory and giant cells (see Fig. 3–9). The exact cause in unknown. Like granulation tissue, it is part of the active process of chronic otitis media with or without otorrhea and may be viewed through a tympanic membrane perforation (yellow-brown chicken fat appearance) or identified at surgery for chronic otitis media. Cholesterin granuloma behind an intact tympanic membrane results in a condition previously described on the basis of appearance as "idiopathic hemotympanum."

Otitis Media and Hearing Loss

In otitis media, all three types of hearing loss (conductive, sensorineural, and mixed) may occur, although the most common hearing loss is conductive in nature. There are multiple causes for the resulting hearing loss:

Conductive hearing loss
  Middle ear effusion
  Ossicular erosion
  Ossicular fixation
  Tympanic membrane perforation
  Fibrosis of middle ear muscles
  Space filling tissues (e.g., granulation tissue, cholesteatoma)
Sensorineural hearing loss
  Hair cell damage (permanent)
  Probably audiologic evidence of round window stiffness (temporary)

An important consequence of hearing loss in preschool years is the deleterious effect of the hearing impairment on language acquisition, academic achievement, and psychosocial development. Although there are no conclusive studies to prove the degree to which these most important sociologic and psychologic problems occur, available studies stress the importance of early identification, prevention, and treatment of the disease. Treatment includes medical and surgical modalities as well as educational intervention as required.

Treatment

There are many "cook books" available that make the treatment of otitis media seem simple; however, as complicated as the disease process itself, treatment can, at times, be quite complex. There is not universal formula for treatment, and whatever therapeutic regimen is used, it should be tailored to a particular patient. Medical treatment most commonly includes antibiotics, antihistamines, decongestants, anti-inflammatory agents, eustachian tube ventilation exercises, and allergic hyposensitization.

PURULENT OTITIS MEDIA

Antimicrobials are definitely indicated in patients with acute purulent otitis media. It has been suggested that the patient be followed without antimicrobial treatment, based on the theory that early treatment of otitis media with antimicrobials reduces the host immunobiologic response to the disease process, resulting in a higher incidence of persistent middle ear effusion and recurrent purulent otitis media. Antimicrobials, however, have significantly reduced the complications of acute purulent otitis media and their use in treating this disease remains the standard of practice. Antimicrobial selection should be based on the known microbiology of the disease. At the time of this writing, S. pneumoniae, H. influenzae, and S. pyogenes are the predominant microorganisms in all age groups and ampicillin or its more convenient congener, amoxicillin, are the antibiotics of choice.

Trimethoprim-sulfa combinations are also gaining popularity for treatment of patients allergic to penicillin and as a drug of choice for all patients with acute purulent otitis media. Patient compliance is good with the twice daily dosage, and the micro-organisms of acute purulent otitis media, including ampicillin-resistant *H. influenzae*, are sensitive to trimethoprim-sulfa in almost 95 per cent of cases. Other antimicrobials of value include erythromycin or erthyromycin-sulfonamide combinations in patients with penicillin allergy and second generation cephalosporins (e.g., cefaclor) for treating ampicillin-resistant *H. influenzae*. Antimicrobials (e.g., penicillin G, sulfonamides, ampicillin) may also be used as prophylaxis in patients with recurrent acute purulent otitis media (three episodes in a 6-month period or four episodes in a 12-month period). Analgesics and antipyretics should be prescribed when indicated.

Myringotomy is employed in the treatment of acute purulent otitis media if the condition does not respond to antimicrobials within 72 to 96 hours, pain is severe, or complications occur (e.g., facial nerve paralysis, meningitis). Culture and sensitivity tests should be obtained at the time of myringotomy. Routine myringotomy in the treatment of acute purulent otitis media is not without hazard and has been shown experimentally not to alter the course of the disease.

Oral preparations of antihistamines and decongestants were widely used in patients with otitis media because they were thought to improve eustachian tube function. Although these preparations should theoretically help in the treatment of otitis media caused by allergy, recent studies have shown that they provide little or no therapeutic benefit and may even decrease eustachian tube function. Systemic decongestants may result in hyperactivity, and antihistamines may cause drowsiness or hyperactivity, especially in children. For these reasons, oral antihistamines and decongestants should not be routinely prescribed for treatment of otitis media. Although topical decongestants in the forms of nasal sprays or drops do reduce mucosal swelling and may be helpful, prolonged use (more than 4 to 5 days) may cause irritation of the nasal mucosa and may result in a condition known as rhinitis medicomentosum. Therefore, these medications should be prescribed with care, and the importance of limiting usage to 4 or 5 days should be carefully explained to the patient.

Although tympanostomy tubes have no place in the treatment of acute purulent otitis media, they can serve as prophylaxis in patients with recurrent acute purulent otitis media if the tubes are placed during a disease-free interval. Recent clinical studies report that the benefits of tympanostomy tubes are significantly greater than those of prophylactic antimicrobials in the treatment of this condition.

SEROUS OTITIS MEDIA AND MUCOID OTITIS MEDIA

Serous otitis media and mucoid otitis media will be discussed together, since their therapies are essentially the same. Reports on hearing loss associated with serous otitis media and mucoid otitis media confirm that it is significant enough to result in psychosocial and educational handicaps if not properly treated. Exercises to help ventilate the middle ear, such as the Valsalva maneuver and politzerization are useful and are recommended as noninvasive forms of therapy.

Systemic antihistamines and decongestants are the most popular forms of therapy for these two conditions, despite the lack of evidence of their therapeutic efficacy and despite their potential for further decreasing eustachian tube function. As such, systemic antihistamines and decongestants are probably not indicated in the treatment of serous otitis media and mucoid otitis media.

The mainstay of treatment of persistent serous otitis media and mucoid otitis media is the placement of tympanostomy tubes. Recent investigations, both clinical and in experimental animals, suggest that the benefits of this form of treatment (immediate improvement in hearing and reduction in the incidence of recurrent acute purulent otitis media and its sequelae) outweigh its potential detriments (risks of anesthesia and surgery and tympanic membrane scarring). The financial impact of tympanostomy-tube insertion is probably no greater than that of the nonsurgical care of the otitis-prone patient, and for these reasons the use of tympanostomy tubes in patients with serous otitis media and mucoid otitis media that has persisted for 2 to 3 months appears efficacious. While tympanostomy tubes are in place, water should be kept out of the external auditory canal, since it can cause infection. Ear protection may be obtained by using petroleum jelly and cotton or by the use of preformed or custom made earplugs.

The use of antimicrobials in the treatment of persistent serous otitis media and mucoid otitis media has been suggested and, based on the microbiology of these two diseases (approximately 35 per cent of effusions are culture positive), this form of therapy appears to have merit. The choice of antimicrobials for the treatment of mucoid and serous otitis media is identical to that for acute purulent otitis media. The drugs should be continued for a duration of 4 to 6 weeks.

Recent reports have suggested that prednisone be used for persistent serous otitis media and mucoid otitis media, which represent inflammatory conditions of the middle ear. Although early studies concerning this form of therapy have been promising, its long-term effects are unknown. Although there is no proof of its effectiveness, allergic hyposensitization seems to help in certain cases of identified hypersensitivity and is worth trying.

Tonsillectomy, with or without adenoidectomy, is another controversial form of treatment for persistent serous otitis media and mucoid otitis media. Current evidence indicates that adenoidectomy in conjunction with tympanostomy tube insertion will reduce the recurrence of middle ear effusion following tympanostomy tube extrusion. The question as to whether or not this reduction in recurrence is significant enough to justify the added risks of this procedure remains unanswered. There is no place for tonsillectomy alone or in combination with adenoidectomy in the treatment of serous otitis media and mucoid otitis media.

CHRONIC OTITIS MEDIA

Otitis media with intractable tissue abnormalities has a mixed bacterial flora. Beacuse of the nature of the bacterial flora and the disease state itself, systemic antibiotics are indicated only when particular soft tissues are infected. In such cases, the drugs of choice are those agents active against *S. pyogenes* and penicillinase-positive staphylococcus. It is most important to recognize that chronic otitis media represents a structural defect in the middle ear cleft, which can be remedied only by surgery. When tympanic membrane perforation is present and active inflammation is apparent (e.g., otorrhea, granulation tissue, erythematous mucosa), topical therapy is indicated as a temporary measure for preoperative preparation and to prevent intracranial extension.

Topical therapy should include mechanical debridement, cleansing and drying, and the application of antiseptics, acidifying agents, antimicrobials, and, in the case of granulation tissue, steroids. Effective topical antimicrobials include aminoglycosides, polymyxins, and chloramphenicol. Many of these agents are theoretically ototoxic when in contact with the round window membrane. However, because clinical occurrence of this complication is not well documented, they remain the standard of care.

BIBLIOGRAPHY

Anson, B. J., and Donaldson, J. A.: Surgical Anatomy of the Temporal Bone and Ear. Philadelphia, W. B. Saunders Co., 1973.

Bluestone, C. D., Paradise, J. L., and Berry, O. C.: Physiology of eustachian tube in the pathogenesis and management of middle ear effusions. Laryngology 82:1654–1670, 1972.

Juhn, S. K., Paparella, M. M., Goycoolea, M. V., et al.: Pathogenesis of otitis media. Ann Otol Rhinol Laryngol 86:481–492, 1977.

Klein, J. L.: Epidemiology of otitis media—otitis media. Publication of the Second National Conference on Otitis Media. Scottsdale, Arizona, March, 1978, pp. 18–20.

Lim, D. J.: Functional morphology of the mucosa of the middle ear and eustachian tube. Ann Otol Rhinol Laryngol 85:36–43, 1976.

Meyerhoff, W. L.: Use of tympanostomy tubes in otitis media. Ann Otol Rhinol Laryngol 90:537–542, 1981.

Meyerhoff, W. L., and Giebink, G. S.: Pathology and microbiology of otitis media. Laryngoscope 92:273–277, 1982.

Meyerhoff, W. L., Paparella, M. M., and Kim, C. S.: Pathology of chronic otitis media. Ann Otol Rhinol Laryngol 87:749–760, 1978.

Meyerhoff, W. L., Paparella, M. M. Oda, M., and Shea, D.: Mycotic infections of the inner ear. Laryngoscope 89:1725–1734, 1979.

Paradise, J. L.: Medical treatment of acute otitis media: a critical essay. Publication of the Second National Conference on Otitis Media. Scottsdale, Arizona, 1978, pp. 79–84.

Sade, J., and Eliezer, N.: Secretory otitis media and the nature of the mucociliary system. Acta Otol 70:351–357, 1970.

William L. Meyerhoff
Stephen Liston
Robert G. Anderson

4

SENSORINEURAL HEARING LOSS

As mentioned in earlier chapters, sensorineural hearing loss is a sign or symptom of underlying disease and usually requires a thorough evaluation in order to make a diagnosis. Treatment directed toward identified etiologies will, on occasion, reverse the hearing loss and correct the underlying disease state. For those cases refractory to medical or surgical treatment, auditory amplification and rehabilitation are extremely useful.

Although it is true that the incidence of sensorineural hearing loss increases markedly with advancing age, the diagnosis of presbycusis or idiopathic sensorineural hearing loss is made far too frequently in the absence of a thorough evaluation. Fortunately, federal regulations now exist to ensure that the patient will be informed about the importance of a medical examination prior to hearing aid acquisition. This law was passed in an effort to protect patients in whom sensorineural hearing loss is a manifestation of a potentially treatable disease.

Sensorineural hearing loss has a legion of etiologies, some local, some regional, and others systemic. The scope of the problem, therefore, necessitates a thorough history and a complete head and neck examination. One must determine the age of onset, mode of progression, presence or absence of fluctuation, bilaterality, and family history. Additional history of ototoxic drugs, otorrhea, head trauma, noise exposure, vertigo, gait disturbance, tinnitus, visual disturbance, otalgia, aural fullness, diplacusis, and recruitment should be sought. The patient should be asked to offer information concerning precipitating events and signs and symptoms of hypothyroidism, multiple scle-

rosis, blood dyscrasias, arteriosclerotic vascular disease, allergy, diabetes mellitus, congenital and acquired neurosensory syphilis, and renal disease.

A comprehensive head and neck examination should emphasize visual inspection of the auricle, external auditory canal, and tympanic membrane. Tympanic membrane mobility should be assessed with the pneumatic otoscope. Tuning fork tests and noise threshold tests will help quantify the hearing loss and establish the site of lesion. It is also important to evaluate the integrity of the cranial nerves and balance system with a neurologic examination. In addition to a careful head and neck examination, further physical examination should include those systems determined to be relative by the history and the differential diagnosis, such as the integument and the cardiovascular, neuromuscular, respiratory, skeletal, and genitourinary systems (see Chapter 1).

Following the history and physical examination, audiologic confirmation of the hearing loss, with special site-of-lesion tests, when applicable, should be obtained. The diagnosis is usually evident by this point in the diagnostic sequence, precluding additional laboratory and radiologic studies. However, if the diagnosis remains obscure, a complete blood count, urinalysis, thyroid function studies, glucose tolerance test, blood clotting studies, lipid fractionation, fluorescent treponemal antibody absorption (FTA-abs) test, and measurement of serum electrolytes with calcium and phosphorus may help elucidate the underlying cause. The physician should perform roentgenographic evaluation of the internal auditory meatus and vestibular studies, especially when faced with unilateral unexplained sensorineural hearing loss. Young patients in whom a syndrome complex is suspected but not obvious should have an electrocardiogram (Jervell and Lange-Nielsen syndrome) and thiocyanate flush (Pendred's syndrome), urinalysis, and creatinine clearance tests performed (Alport's syndrome).

Etiology

Etiologies for sensorineural hearing loss are numerous and can best be understood if classified in an orderly manner. Sensorineural hearing loss may be genetic or nongenetic. Genetic disorders imply association with reproduction or inheritance, whereas nongenetic disorders usually result from environmental factors. Regardless of whether a disorder is genetic or nongenetic, it may manifest as a congenital problem (present at birth) or be delayed in its presentation. As a result, there are two basic categories of sensorineural hearing loss and two subcategories (see Tables 1–6 to 1–9).

CONGENITAL SENSORINEURAL HEARING LOSS

Sensorineural hearing loss that is present at birth is said to be congenital. It may be the result of environmental or genetic factors. Brainstem response audiometry now allows objective auditory testing in children as young as 6 weeks of age. Therefore, children suspected of having a hearing loss and those children in a particularly high-risk category should be examined as soon as possible to avoid the sequelae attendant to congenital hearing loss with delayed diagnosis and treatment (see Chapter 9).

Genetic

Genetic congenital sensorineural hearing loss may occur alone or as part of a syndrome. Often there is some form of inner ear anatomic abnormality accounting for the sensorineural hearing loss, and these anatomic abnormalities may be divided into four basic categories, depending on their severity (Michel's aplasia Mondini's dysplasia, Scheibe's deafness and Bing-Siebenmann's deafness). These inner ear abnormalities may coexist with middle ear abnormalities, adding a conductive component to the hearing loss. Although surgical intervention may be of benefit for the con-

ductive component, the sensorineural hearing loss usually requires amplification.

Inner Ear Anatomic Abnormalities. In Michel's aplasia, there is total absence of the bony labyrinth and membranous labyrinth. This rare condition is transmitted by an autosomal dominant gene, and owing to the severity of the deformity, the patients are totally deaf. The diagnosis may be suspected following temporal bone polytomography, although a similar roentgenographic picture may occur with labyrinthitis ossificans, in which the entire inner ear is replaced by bone due to osteoneogenesis (see Fig. 3–14).

In Mondini's dysplasia, there is a partial aplasia of the bony labyrinth and membranous labyrinth. In this disorder, the cochlea has one and one half turns, with the middle and apical turns coalescing to form a common space, the scala communis. The normal cochlea contains two and one half turns (Fig. 4–1). This autosomal dominant malformation may also have attendant abnormalities within the vestibular system. The associated hearing loss varies in severity and may be of little significance.

Scheibe's deafness is usually inherited as an autosomal recessive trait and is the most common form of genetic congenital sensorineural hearing loss. Anatomically this disorder causes abnormal development of the saccule and cochlear duct (Fig. 4–2). Although most patients with this condition are deaf, some demonstrate hearing in the low frequencies.

Bing-Siebenmann's deafness is also an inherited malformation. There is partial aplasia of the cochlear duct (especially at the basal turn), which results in a high-frequency hearing loss.

As mentioned previously, these inner ear abnormalities may occur alone or as part of a syndrome associated with other abnormalities. The recognition of these syndromes is extremely important if one is to provide proper genetic counseling and early amplification. Medical and surgical therapies usually do not help these conditions and will be mentioned only when they have been shown to be beneficial.

Syndromes. Congenital genetic sensorineural hearing loss may be associated with external ear abnormalities. This association is seen in the otofacial cervical syndrome, an autosomal dominant disease and the syndrome of cervical fistulae, preauricular pits, and autosomal dominant mixed hearing loss. Lop ears have also been associated with

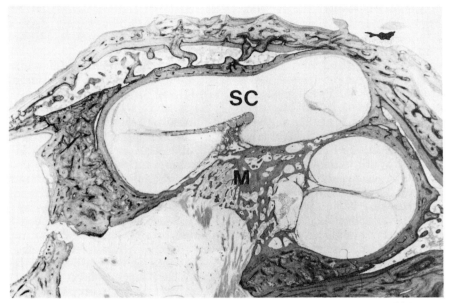

Figure 4–1. Mondini's deformity. M = modiolous; SC = scala communis. (× 20.)

congenital genetic sensorineural hearing loss (see Fig. 1–2).

In other syndromes, sensorineural hearing loss may be associated with eye disease; Usher's syndrome is the most common of these, accounting for 3 to 15 per cent of profoundly deaf children. Patients with this syndrome, which is inherited by an autosomal recessive gene, have retinitis pigmentosa and sensorineural hearing loss.

Congenital genetic sensorineural hearing loss and musculoskeletal disease may also coexist. Apert's syndrome is inherited by a dominant gene and includes congenital sensorineural hearing loss, frontal bossing, exophthalmus, hypoplastic maxilla, and syn-

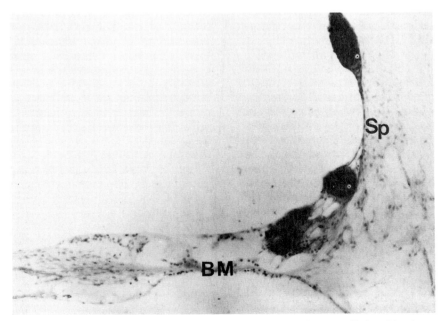

Figure 4–2. Scheibe's deafness. The cochlear duct is collapsed onto spiral ligament (Sp) and basilar membrane (BM). (× 300.)

dactyly (see Fig. 2–6). Apert's syndrome occurs in 1 in 160,000 births, but because of the neonatal mortality rate, it is present only in about 1 in 2,000,000 members of the population. Marfan's syndrome is also inherited by a dominant gene and is characterized by pigeon breast, dolichocephaly, hammer toes, and congenital sensorineural hearing loss. Patients with the dominant syndromes of Pierre Robin and Crouzon also display facial and skull deformities. Patients with Pierre Robin syndrome present with glossoptosis, micrognathia, and cleft palate. Crouzon's disease is characterized by premature fusion of the cranial sutures, shallow orbits, exophthalmus, parrot nose, hypoplastic maxilla, and sensorineural hearing loss.

Congenital genetic sensorineural hearing loss is also observed in disorders of pigmentation. Patients with Waardenburg's syndrome, described in 1951, present with a broad nasal root, confluent eyebrows, heterochromic irides, white forelock, and congenital deafness in one or both ears. This disorder accounts for about 2 to 3 per cent of congenitally deaf patients. Waardenburg's syndrome is divided into two varieties: that with dystopia canthorum (Type I) and that without dystopia canthorum (Type II).

Albinism, another disorder in pigmentation, can also be associated with sensorineural hearing loss. An additional syndrome combining abnormalities in pigmentation and sensorineural hearing loss is the leopard syndrome, which is inherited as an autosomal dominant gene. Leopard syndrome is characterized by lentigines, electrocardiogram (EKG) abnormalities, pulmonary artery stenosis, abnormalities of the genitalia, retardation of growth, and sensorineural deafness in 25 per cent of cases.

Congenital genetic sensorineural hearing loss frequently is seen in association with nervous system disorders. Mental retardation is one of the more frequent conditions associated with genetic sensorineural hearing loss. Ataxia is also found in conjunction with this type of hearing loss in a number of syndromes. Other neurologic phenomena such as myoclonic epilepsy, sensory neuropathies, and neural paralyses are found in combination with hearing loss.

Congenital genetic sensorineural hearing loss is also seen in patients with thyroid disease. Pendred first called attention to the syndrome that bears his name. Pendred's syndrome is characterized by goiter and bilateral congenital sensorineural hearing loss.

The goiter occurs at an early age, but the patients are usually euthyroid. Pendred's syndrome is inherited as an autosomal recessive trait, and it occurs in from 1 to 7.5 per 100,000 live births. The goiter is due to an enzymatic defect in the organic binding of iodine in the course of thyroxine synthesis, which accounts for the positive perchlorate or thiocyanate test findings in these patients. The decrease in organic binding results in an increase in thyroid-stimulating hormone and subsequent goiter.

Congenital genetic sensorineural hearing loss and abnormalities in cardiac conduction were first reported in 1957 by Jervell and Lange-Nielsen. They described a syndrome of sensorineural hearing loss, prolonged Q–T interval on EKG, and attacks of syncope with occasional sudden death. This syndrome is inherited as an autosomal recessive trait and occurs in three to four per million live births.

Congenital genetic sensorineural hearing loss has also been associated with several chromosomal abnormalities such as Turner's syndrome and trisomies 21, 13, and 18 (Fig. 4–3).

Nongenetic

Nongenetic congenital sensorineural hearing loss is usually the result of intrauterine (prenatal) or perinatal insult.

Prenatal Causes. One of the most common prenatal causes of deafness used to be maternal rubella. The rubella virus crosses the placenta to produce congenital abnormalities in the growing fetus. The rubella triad consists of congenital cataracts, deafness, and heart disease. The availability of an effective vaccine against rubella has greatly reduced the number of such "rubella babies." Toxoplasmosis and syphilis are other infections that can cross the placenta and cause hearing loss in the newborn.

Endemic cretinism is associated with a 70 per cent incidence of cogenital sensorineural hearing loss. The hearing loss has been attributed to both slow mentation and anatomic abnormalities of the cerebral cortex, middle ear, and petrous portion of the temporal bone. Thyroid therapy is of little value in restoration of hearing but is necessary to reduce the mental retardation.

Ototoxic drugs given to the mother during the gestational period may also cross the placental barrier to produce congenital sensorineural hearing loss. Perhaps the most infamous of these drugs is thalidomide, which frequently produced a congenital hearing loss along with many other congenital deformities.

Perinatal Causes. Anoxia from such causes as abruptio placentae, umbilical cord compression, or complicated delivery may result in sensorineural hearing loss. Intracranial hemorrhage due to a complicated delivery is another potential cause. Premature infants are at greater risk for hearing loss than are term infants.

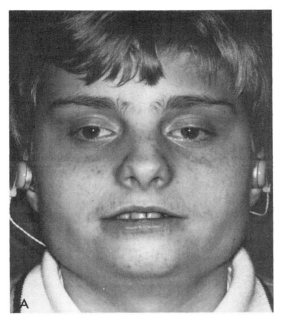

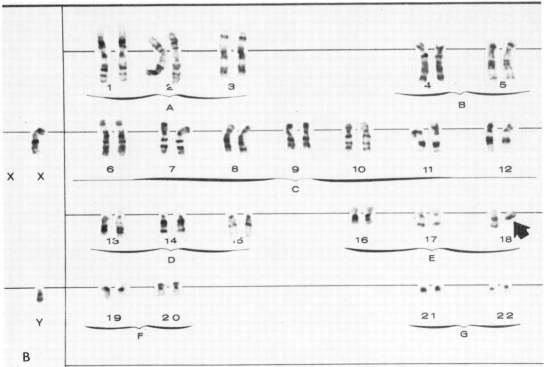

Figure 4–3. *A,* Facial appearance and *(B)* karyotype of a patient with deletion of long arm of chromosome 18. (Courtesy of Drs. Jarosian Cervenka and Karlin Moller.)

Kernicterus (the deposition of a brown pigment in the basal ganglia and cochlear nuclei) often results in sensorineural hearing loss. This condition is due to an abnormally elevated level of circulating nonconguated bilirubin and usually occurs owing to the destruction of the infant's erythrocytes by a maternal antibody caused by Rh incompatibility. The hearing loss can be prevented by exchange transfusions, ultraviolet phototherapy, or phenobarbital therapy to lower the circulating bilirubin level. RhoGAM is an agent that prevents maternal sensitization to the Rh antibody, and it should decrease the number of infants at risk in the future.

DELAYED SENSORINEURAL HEARING LOSS

A wide variety of postnatal environmental factors contribute to acquired sensorineural hearing loss. However, in addition, certain genetic traits also give rise to sensorineural hearing loss that manifests later in life.

Genetic

Genetic sensorineural hearing loss that develops with time may occur alone (isolated) or be associated with a syndrome. The hearing loss may be present early in life or may not become evident until the patient matures. The frequency range of the hearing loss may be confined to the low, middle, or high frequencies and the unilateral or bilateral loss may be stable or progress with age. Treatment of the sensorineural hearing loss is usually in the form of amplification.

Isolated. The two most frequent genetic causes of progressive sensorineural hearing loss are cochlear otosclerosis and progressive familial sensorineural hearing loss. Otosclerosis is a primary disease of the labyrinthine capsule, transmitted, in most cases, by an autosomal dominant gene. Histologically, otosclerosis occurs in up to 10 per cent of the population although less than 10 per cent of affected individuals manifest this disorder clinically. The sites of predilection are the fissula ante fenestram (just anterior to the stapes footplate) and the fossula post fenestram (just posterior to the stapes footplate), resulting in fixation of the stapes and an insidious, progressive, conductive hearing loss. The conductive aspect of the disease is discussed in Chapter 2.

Otosclerosis, because of cochlear involvement, may also result in sensorineural hearing loss. Various explanations for this occurrence have been offered. Some observers suggest that the otosclerotic focus produces an ototoxic substance that enters the arterial circulation of the cochlea, whereas others propose that the otosclerotic focus shunts blood away from the cochlear end organ, resulting in ischemia. Morphologic alterations of the cochlea have also been identified with cochlear otosclerosis and are thought by some to be the main cause of the associated sensorineural hearing loss (Fig. 4–4).

The diagnosis of cochlear otosclerosis should be considered in patients with stapedial otosclerosis who develop a sensorineural hearing loss. These patients usually have a family history of otosclerosis and may also have a positive Schwartze's sign (red blush on promontory when viewed with the otoscope). This red blush is thought to be secondary to increased vascularity in the area of the stapes footplate. Tomographic evidence of cochlear otosclerosis may be obtained, but there appears to be a high incidence of false-negative and false-positive examination results. The exact incidence of cochlear otosclerosis and whether or not it occurs in the absence of stapedial involvement are not known. Suggested treatment includes sodium fluoride (40 to 60 mg per day), calcium carbonate (10 gm per day), and vitamin D (400 units per day). There is strong evidence that this treatment reduces or altogether stops the progression of the sensorineural hearing loss.

Progressive familial sensorineural hearing loss may occur early or late in life as an isolated entity and is a major cause of delayed sensorineural hearing loss. It frequently goes undiagnosed, however, and is often mistakenly labeled idiopathic or presbycusis even when seen in relatively young individuals. The audiometric pattern may either be sloping in the high frequencies (Fig. 4–5) or concave, with the greatest losses being in the middle frequencies. A careful family history will often lead to the diagnosis. The mode of transmission may be dominant, recessive, or X-linked and, aside from amplification and lip-reading education, no other therapy is effective.

Syndromes. In addition to occurring as an isolated entity, progressive sensorineural hearing loss occurs as part of several known syndromes. Delayed genetic sensorineural hearing loss may occur in association with eye disease. Alstrom's syndrome combines retinal degeneration with diabetes mellitus,

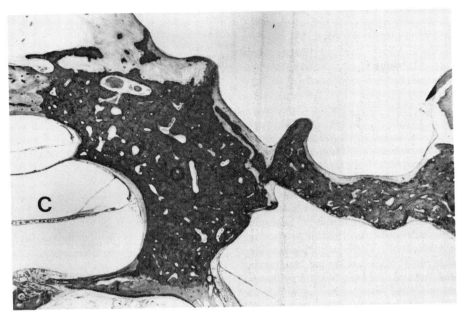

Figure 4–4. Cochlear otosclerosis. C = cochlea; O = otosclerosis. (× 30.)

obesity, and sensorineural hearing loss. It is inherited through a recessive gene, and the patients develop nystagmus and visual loss secondary to retinal degeneration at about 1 year of age. The hearing loss is progressive and begins just prior to adolescence, with diabetes mellitus usually presenting soon after adolescence.

Refsum's syndrome is of interest because it can be diagnosed by amniocentesis. This syndrome is characterized by retinitis pigmentosa, hypertrophic peripheral neuropathy, ataxia, and progressive sensorineural hearing loss. It is due to an enzymatic defect,

which results in an accumulation of phytanic acid. The condition may be improved somewhat by a diet low in phytol and phytanic acid. The mode for genetic inheritance is recessive.

Other syndromes involving genetic delayed sensorineural hearing loss and eye disease are those in which optic atrophy, myopia, and/or blue sclera are associated with sensorineural hearing loss. Corneal dystrophies and degenerations as well as ophthalmoplegias are also seen with sensorineural hearing loss. Cockayne's syndrome is inherited as an autosomal recessive trait

Figure 4–5. Pure tone audiogram. Audiometric pattern of high-frequency hearing loss.

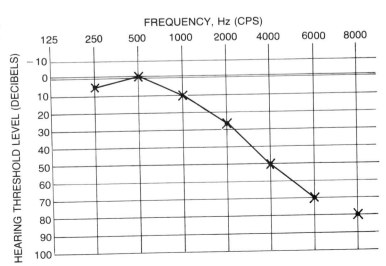

and is characterized by dwarfism, mental retardation, retinal degeneration, and delayed sensorineural hearing loss.

Delayed genetic sensorineural hearing loss is seen in a number of syndromes displaying musculoskeletal disorders. These disorders include bony dysplasias, which range in severity from those involving only a few bones to those involving the entire skeleton. Joint fusions may also be associated with sensorineural hearing loss. Examples of musculoskeletal disease and sensorineural hearing loss include Paget's disease, osteogenesis imperfecta, Albers-Schönberg disease, and Klippel-Feil anomaly (fusion of the cervical vertebrae).

Paget's is an uncommon disease, primarily occurring in elderly males and associated with hearing loss in a large percentage of patients. Paget's disease causes considerable deformation of the skull (including the temporal bone in advanced lesions) with associated arteriovenous shunting. It is a chronic, progressive, and nonfatal disease of bone, characterized by active resorption and irregular reconstruction with hypertrophied, vascular, demineralized bone. The histologic picture is quite similar to that of otosclerosis. The hearing loss is usually mixed or purely sensorineural. Ossicular fixation is responsible for the conductive component. The same etiologies suggested to be responsible for the sensorineural component of otosclerosis are also proposed as the causes of the sensorineural hearing loss in Paget's disease. The mode of inheritance is most likely autosomal dominant, with incomplete penetrance and variable expressivity. Calcitonin has been used to treat Paget's disease, but its effect on the hearing loss is still uncertain. Juvenile Paget's disease (hyperphosphatasia) is also associated with sensorineural hearing loss.

The syndrome of osteogenesis imperfecta (van der Hoevede Kleyn syndrome) is congenital in 10 per cent and "tarda" in the remaining 90 per cent of patients. Although complete deafness is rarely observed, impaired hearing is present in 30 to 90 per cent patients with the tarda type. The hearing loss is often considered to be conductive and symmetrical but may be mixed or purely sensorineural. It usually becomes clinically evident by the third decade of life, progressing, in some individuals, to profound or rarely total deafness. Stapedectomy may eliminate the conductive component of the hearing loss, but amplification is the only available therapy for the sensorineural component. Osteogenesis imperfecta is a hereditary disorder, most likely inherited as an autosomal dominant with variable expressivity. In addition to hearing loss patients with this disorder present with fragile bones, large skulls, blue sclera, triangular faces, and hemorrhagic tendencies.

Hearing loss caused by stenosis of the internal auditory canal and occasional ossicular abnormalities is also a feature of Albers-Schönberg disease (osteopetrosis). Hearing loss may also be found with Klippel-Feil anomaly.

Several syndromes are characterized by the association of renal disease with acquired sensorineural hearing loss. The most important of these is Alport's disease, which is probably inherited as heterogeneity (a single phenotype resulting from more than one genotype). Alport's disease accounts for about 1 per cent of genetic deafness. The syndrome is characterized by hematuria, albuminuria, and pyuria. These urinary findings usually occur in the early teens or early 20s and result in hypertension and renal failure. Males are much more severely affected than females. The hearing loss begins in the late teens or early 20s and, like the renal manifestations, is worse in males. Renal transplantation has been able to help the renal problem and in some cases, has been able to improve the sensorineural hearing levels.

Inherited disorders of mucopolysaccharide metabolism are often associated with inherited acquired sensorineural hearing loss. Hurler's syndrome, Hunter's syndrome, Sanfillippo's syndrome, and the syndromes of Morquio and Maroteaux-Lamy all occur in conjunction with hearing loss. Hurler's syndrome, inherited as an autosomal recessive trait, is characterized by failure to grow, mental retardation, coarse facial features, and corneal clouding. Hunter's syndrome, which is very similar to Hurler's syndrome, is due to an X-linked gene. Mannosidosis may also be associated with sensorineural deafness.

Lastly, there is a syndrome in which delayed genetic sensorineural hearing loss occurs with tumor formation. Von Recklinghausen's syndrome is inherited as an autosomal dominant trait or through spontaneous mutation and produces progressive sensorineural hearing loss as the result of cerebellopontine angle neoplasms. These neoplasms are usually acoustic neuromas, although meningiomas may occur. The treatment, surgical removal of the neoplasms, rarely improves or even maintains the preoperative hearing level. Total hearing loss is often present before surgery and is almost always present following surgery.

Nongenetic

A multitude of environmental factors have an adverse effect on the auditory system and, with time, result in sensorineural hearing loss.

Trauma. Trauma causes hearing loss in a variety of ways. Perhaps the best known and most common mechanism is noise-induced hearing loss, although sensorineural hearing loss may also result from temporal bone fractures, penetrating injuries, and sudden barometric pressure changes.

The most preventable sensorineural hearing loss at the present time is the insidious loss associated with exposure to loud noises. The term noise-induced hearing loss is used to describe a hearing loss that follows a long period of exposure to loud noises, whereas acoustic trauma refers to the hearing loss caused by a single exposure to an extremely intense noise, such as an explosion. Exposure to noise initially produces a temporary hearing threshold shift, with further exposure resulting in a permanent threshold shift. Initially, this hearing loss characteristically involves the frequency range around 4000 Hz, although with continued noise exposure, the hearing loss becomes more severe and spreads out to also include adjacent frequencies. Currently, the most widely accepted theory concerning noise-induced hearing loss is that relating to total energy presented to the ear. Basically, this theory states that shorter noise exposure at high intensity cause amounts of damage similar to longer periods of exposure at less intensity. The minimum noise level known to cause noise-induced hearing loss regardless of duration is about 80 to 85 dB. Histologically, structural damage to the hair cells and stria vascularis is identified with noise exposure.

It has been known for many years that workers in noisy industries are prone to develop hearing loss, but it has been only recently that legislation has mandated the legal limit of noise exposure to which a worker may be subjected. There are no medications that will protect against noise-induced hearing loss, and since the hair cells themselves are destroyed, the hearing loss is irreversible (Fig. 4–6). Ear protection against noise is the most effective preventative measure available. Vitamin A and other proposed therapies for noise-induced hearing loss are not of proven value.

Fractures involving the labyrinth or internal auditory canal often result in sensorineural hearing loss (see Figs. 2–10 and 2–11). Traditionally, temporal bone fractures

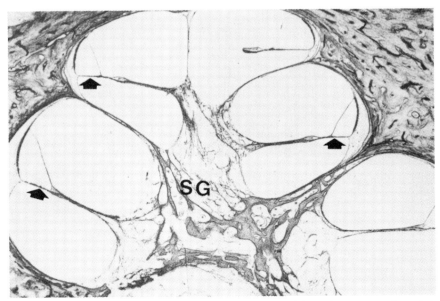

Figure 4–6. Acoustic trauma, with loss of the organ of Corti (arrows) and loss of neurons in the spiral ganglion (SG). (× 20.)

are classified as longitudinal or transverse. Longitudinal fractures are usually associated with a conductive hearing loss due to disarticulation of the ossicular chain. Transverse fractures actually involve the labyrinth or internal auditory canal and result in sensorineural hearing loss. Blows to the head that do not produce a skull fracture may also cause a sensorineural hearing loss resembling the hearing loss seen in acoustic trauma.

A variety of penetrating injuries, including surgery, can be associated with sensorineural hearing loss. Occasionally patients who introduce objects through the tympanic membrane (e.g., cotton-tip applicators) will displace the stapes into the vestibule and cause sensorineural hearing loss. High-velocity missle wounds to the temporal bone may also be responsible for sensorineural hearing loss. Opening into the perilymphatic space during surgical procedures may result in partial or total sensorineural hearing loss.

Sudden changes in barometric pressure, such as those associated with flying, underwater diving, and sneezing or coughing may rupture the round window membrane or oval window anulus. These injuries result in a sensorineural hearing loss and frequently vertigo. If treated promptly, these fistulae can be repaired surgically with return of hearing. Another type of pressure change associated with hearing loss is seen in divers who suffer the bends as a result of a rapid ascent. Nitrogen comes out of solution to form gas emboli within the vascular system. These emboli impact in small blood vessels, resulting in distal ischemia. The treatment is immediate recompression followed by slow decompression.

Ototoxic Agents. There are a variety of drugs known to adversely affect hearing. Only a few, such as aspirin and quinine, cause reversible hearing loss (Table 4–1).

At high doses, salicylates characteristically produce tinnitus. Although they may also be responsible for a sensorineural hearing loss, it is reversible with termination of salicylate therapy. The salicylates are thought to block an enzyme system within the inner ear, resulting in uncoupling of oxidative phosphorylation within the cochlea.

The renal tubule and the stria vascularis have many metabolic similarities. Hence it is not entirely surprising that certain diuretics can cause sensorineural hearing loss. Ethacrynic acid produces a reversible hearing loss at low doses, although the hearing loss may become permanent with doses that are higher than those recommended by the package insert. Pharmacologically, furosemide behaves in a similar fashion, but the development of hearing loss with its administration tends to be idiosyncratic and much less common than with ethacrynic acid.

Quinine can be the cause of temporary or permanent sensorineural hearing loss. It also crosses the placental barrier, resulting in hearing loss in the developing fetus. Hearing loss and tinnitus from quinine are frequently seen in elderly patients who receive this therapy for leg cramps.

Aminoglycoside antibiotics are ototoxic and specifically capable of destroying the hair cells and stria vascularis of the inner ear, resulting in irreversible hearing loss (Fig. 4–7). The degree of ototoxicity is increased by noise exposure and use with other ototoxic drugs. Dihydrostreptomycin, kanamycin, viomycin, and neomycin are particularly toxic to the cochlear hair cells, and streptomycin and gentamicin tend to affect the vestibular hair cells before destroying the cochlear hair cells. Tobramycin, a relatively new addition to the group of aminoglycoside antibiotics, is apparently less toxic to the inner ear than gentamicin. In addition, nethecillin, a new synthetic aminoglycoside, holds promise of being less ototoxic than any of the presently available aminoglycosides. Since the effect of most

Table 4–1. OTOTOXIC AGENTS

Diuretics
Ethacrynic acid
Furosemide
Anti-inflammatory Drugs
Salicylates
Indomethacin
Antimalarials
Quinine
Chloroquine
Antineoplastic Drugs
Nitrogen mustard
Cis-platinum
Aminoglycoside Antibiotics
Streptomycin
Dihydrostreptomycin
Neomycin
Gentamicin
Kanamycin
Tobramycin
Amikacin
Netilmicin
Other Antibiotics
Erythromycin
Vancomycin
Heavy Metals

aminoglycosides is insidious, all these drugs may be partially responsible for hearing loss that becomes apparent only weeks or months after therapy has been discontinued. Early loss can be detected by daily high-frequency audiometry and electronystagmography. The aminoglycosides are excreted by the kidney, and any degree of renal impairment renders a patient much more susceptible to these ototoxic drugs. It should also be noted that aminoglycosides can cross the placental barrier, causing hearing loss in unborn children.

Cytotoxic agents such as nitrogen mustard and especially *cis*-platinum can cause a sensorineural hearing loss. Severe irreversible hearing loss is rarely one of the side effects of serum sickness when the tetanus antitoxin is of equine origin.

Infectious Agents. A large variety of microbes, including viral, bacterial, mycobacterial, spirochetal, and fungal agents, are capable of infecting the labyrinth and destroying its ability to function. Each type of infection has its own particular characteristics.

Viral organisms may result in sensorineural hearing loss by causing perilymphatic labyrinthitis, endolymphatic labyrinthitis, neuronitis, or vasculitis, and in some cases the loss may be quite sudden. Viral infections of the labyrinth may occur as part of a generalized infection or may be localized, with the labyrinth as the only organ involved. The viruses implicated in sensorineural hearing loss include rubella (both prenatal and postnatal), rubeola, mumps, herpes zoster, adenovirus III and other viruses associated with upper respiratory tract infections, the virus of infectious mononucleosis, and cytomegalovirus. Viral infection may involve one or both ears. Mumps typically is responsible for a unilateral sensorineural hearing loss. In children, the loss of hearing in only one ear may not be discovered until a later date, and since the precipitating event has passed, etiologic diagnosis is often impossible. It is hoped that the use of mumps, measles, and rubella vaccines will decrease the number of patients with hearing loss attributable to these viruses.

In general, the histologic findings seen in the temporal bone following a viral labyrinthitis include atrophy of the organ of Corti and stria vascularis and morphologic changes in the tectorial membrane. The ganglion cells may also be involved, and in many cases, Reissner's membrane is collapsed.

Bacterial infections may also involve the inner ear in several ways. Serous labyrinthitis is presumed to be secondary to passage of bacterial toxins from suppurative otitis media across the round or oval windows, with resultant sensorineural hearing loss and vertigo. The diagnosis is usually made in retrospect when the hearing returns to normal after the otitis media resolves. Over the long term, repeated bouts of serous

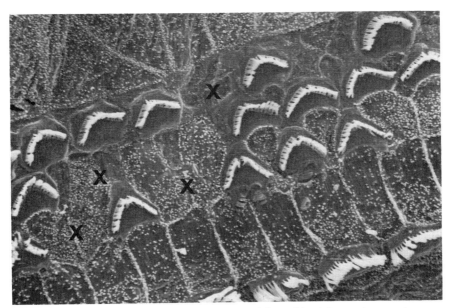

Figure 4–7. Outer hair cell region from the third turn of a chinchilla cochlea following kanamycin exposure. Outer hair cell loss can be seen (X).

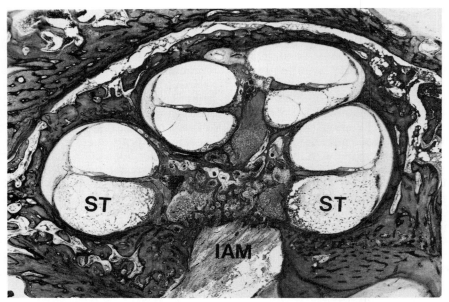

Figure 4–8. Meningogenic suppurative labyrinthitis, with inflammatory fibrosis within the internal auditory meatus (IAM) and scala tympani (ST). (× 20.)

labyrinthitis associated with chronic suppurative or acute recurrent otitis media may lead to a permanent sensorineural hearing loss. These events can usually be prevented by early and adequate medical and surgical treatment of recurrent acute and chronic otitis media.

Suppurative labyrinthitis occurs as a result of bacterial invasion of the labyrinth itself. The route of invasion is usually from the middle ear cavity (tympanogenic) or from the meninges (meningogenic) (Fig. 4–8). In most cases, all labyrinthine function is lost. The labyrinth fills with purulent exudate, and healing takes place by fibrosis or new bone formation (labyrinthitis ossificans) (see Fig. 3–14).

Perilabyrinthitis is another way in which bacterial infection may involve the inner ear. It is associated with a labyrinthine fistula and usually results from erosion of the otic capsule by cholesteatoma or granulation tissue. Osteitis of syphilis used to be a common cause of labyrinthine fistula but is seen infrequently today. Clinically, the presence of a fistula is often accompanied by a positive fistula sign, in which nystagmus is seen following application of pressure to the external auditory canal. The most common location of a cholesteatomatous fistula is the lateral semicircular canal. The fistula may become the route by which the labyrinth is invaded by granulation tissue and fibrous tissue. Perilabyrinthitis is an indication for immediate surgical treatment of the cholesteatoma or chronic otitis media. Considerable skill and judgment are required to best deal with the cholesteatoma matrix over the fistula without jeopardizing the remaining hearing.

Tuberculous labyrinthitis occurs secondary to tuberculous otitis media or tuberculous meningitis. The labyrinthitis develops slowly; therefore the typical signs of labyrinthitis (sensorineural hearing loss and vertigo) may not be prominent. The sensorineural hearing loss is usually overshadowed by the considerable conductive hearing loss seen with tuberculous otitis media. The diagnosis is made from mucosal biopsies and culture of the exudate and granulation tissue. Treatment requires medical control of the tuberculous infection followed by surgical correction of irreversible damage.

The inner ear may be involved by either the acquired or congenital form of syphilis. In the acquired form, the labyrinth may be affected by the acute lymphocytic meningitis of secondary syphilis or the tertiary stage of syphilis. In the latter, the labyrinth is characterized by vasculitis, osteitis, or gumma formation involving the otic capsule.

Congenital syphilis is due to transplacental infection of the fetus and is divided into two types. Patients with the tardive type of congenital syphilis may present with a fluctuating hearing loss and vertigo similar to that of Meniere's disease. They may also present with sudden deafness, which may be profound and bilateral. Hennebert's sign, a positive fistula sign in the absence of a perforated tympanic membrane, was originally described in association with syphilis. This sign is probably caused by adhesions between the saccule and the stapes footplate, which occur with long-standing endolymphatic hydrops. It is necessary to use both serologic tests for syphilis (e.g., Venereal Disease Research Laboratory [VDRL], Kahn, Kline, Kolmar, Rapid plasma reagin) and treponemal antigen tests (*Treponema pallidum* immobilization [TPI], FTA-ABS, microhemagglutination—*Treponema pallidum* [MHA-TP]) to rule out syphilitic hearing loss. After treatment, the VDRL may revert to normal, although spirochetes may persist in a variety of organ systems. Congenital syphilis is treated by a long course of penicillin (some advocate 90 days). Steroids are used to reduce inflammation and may have to be continued for the rest of the patients life to guard against progressive or sudden irreversible sensorineural hearing loss.

Although fungal infections of the inner ear are rare, they have been reported in debilitated patients. Patients with terminal cancer and those being treated with steroids or immunosuppressive drugs are particularly susceptible to this disorder. The fungi reach the inner ear through either the internal auditory canal (meningogenic), vascular system (hematogenic), or middle ear (tympanogenic) and cause progressive and irreversible sensorineural hearing loss (Figs. 4–9 to 4–11).

Neoplasms. Acoustic neuromas are benign tumors derived from Schwann's cells. They are the most common tumors in the posterior cranial fossa, and the usual site of tumor formation is the superior vestibular nerve. In a small number of families, bilateral acoustic neuromas occur and these are generally inherited as part of an autosomal dominant trait (von Recklinghausen's disease).

Acoustic neuromas usually arise within the internal auditory meatus (Fig. 4–12). Tumor growth results in enlargement of the dimensions of the internal auditory meatus, which can be identified radiographically (Fig. 4–13). If untreated, the neuroma will expand into the cerebellopontine angle, producing sensorineural hearing loss (which may occur suddenly), tinnitus, and possibly dysequilibrium. Characteristically, speech discrimination is disproportionately poor in comparison with the pure-tone thresholds. Tone decay and decay of the stapedial acoustic reflex may also occur. Electronystagmography and brainstem response audiometry are frequently abnormal. As the neuroma grows, it impinges on the trigeminal nerve, causing a decrease in the corneal reflex and eventually long tract and cerebellar signs. The level of protein in the perilymph and the cerebrospinal fluid is often elevated, and patients with very large tumors will present with headache and papilledema.

It is axiomatic that every adult patient

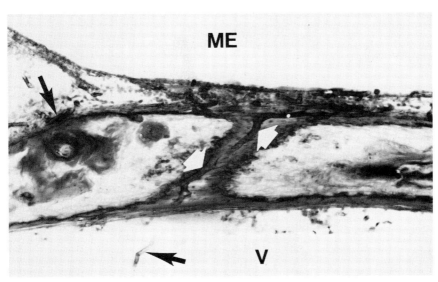

Figure 4–9. Oval window anulus. *Mucor* sp. (arrows) can be identified in the middle ear (ME), vestibule (V), and oval window anulus. (× 150.) (From Meyerhoff, W. L., Paparella, M. M., Oda, M., and Shea, D.: Mycotic infections of the inner ear. Laryngoscope 89:1725–1734, 1979. Reproduced with permission.)

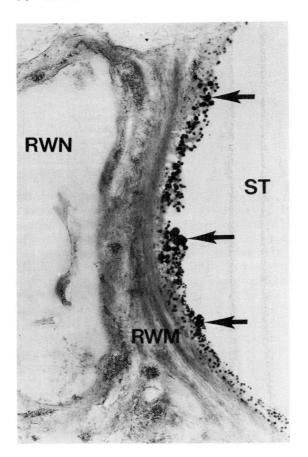

Figure 4–10. Round window membrane (RWM). *Candida* sp. (arrows) can be seen in the scala tympani (ST). There is an amorphous precipitate in the round window niche (RWN). (× 80.) (From Meyerhoff, W. L., Paparella, M. M., Oda, M., and Shea, D.: Mycotic infections of the inner ear. Laryngoscope 89:1725–1734, 1979. Reproduced with permission.)

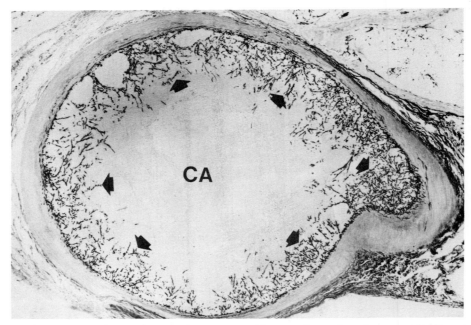

Figure 4–11. Carotid artery (CA) in its temporal bone course. *Mucor* sp. (arrows) can be seen within the artery. (× 25.) (From Meyerhoff, W. L., Paparella, M. M., Oda, M., and Shea D.: Mycotic infections of the inner ear. Laryngoscope 89:1725–1734, 1979. Reproduced with permission.)

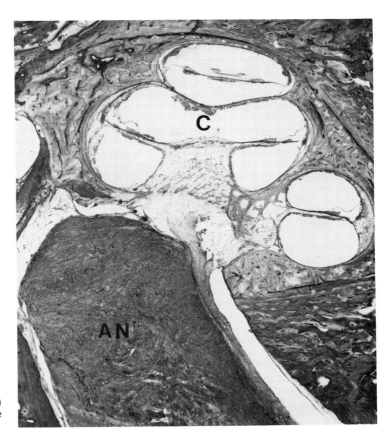

Figure 4–12. Acoustic neuroma (AN) adjacent to the cochlea (C) and filling the internal auditory canal.

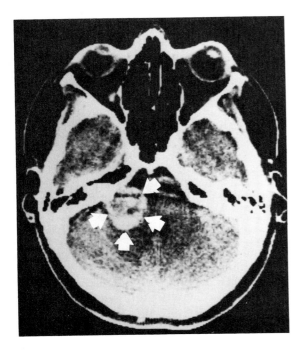

Figure 4–13. Computerized tomogram showing cerebellopontine angle tumor (arrows).

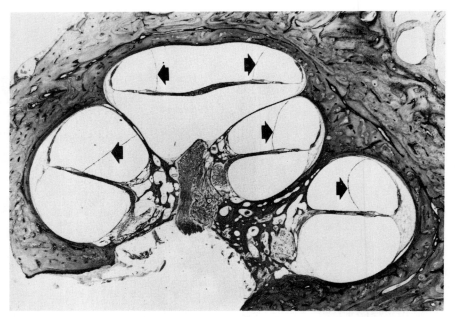

Figure 4–14. Cross section of cochlea showing hydropic changes of Reissner's membrane (arrows).

with unilateral sensorineural hearing loss should be investigated for acoustic neuroma, and it is imperative to diagnose acoustic neuroma early, since small tumors can be removed without damage to the facial nerve and, in some instances, without loss of residual hearing.

Idiopathic. Meniere's disease is characterized histologically by endolymphatic hydrops (Fig. 4–14). Patients complain of intermittent incapacitating vertigo associated with nausea and vomiting. Fluctuating sensorineural hearing loss, tinnitus, and sensation of aural fullness are also characteristics of the disease. Early in the course of the disease, the hearing loss is in the low frequencies; hearing returns almost to normal during remissions. Audiometrically, the site of the lesion is in the cochlea, and recruitment is present. As the attacks continue, the hearing threshold tends to decrease and the high tones tend to be affected as well. The hearing level characteristically improves after a glycerol- or urea-induced diuresis, and this is the basis of a diagnostic test for endolymphatic hydrops. The diagnosis of Meniere's syndrome can be safely made in any patient who manifests fluctuant sensorineural hearing, aural fullness, tinnitus, and episodic vertigo. Since several underlying factors may precipitate this symptom complex, the physician must exclude them by testing the patient for inhalent and food

allergens, syphilis, hypothyroidism, and diabetes mellitus. The incidence of metabolic abnormalities causing Meniere's syndrome appears to be quite low if an association exists at all. This raises the question as to the cost effectiveness of these tests. In the absence of an identifiable etiology, nonspecific therapy should be instituted. Since fluid build-up in the endolymphatic space is characteristic of Meniere's disease, a low salt diet may improve all symptoms. If not, a mild diuretic (e.g., hydrochlorthiazide) may be used. The vertigo and associated nausea and vomiting may be reduced by the use of antihistamines (e.g., meclizine), tranquilizers (e.g., diazepam [Valium]), or anticholinergics (e.g., sublingual or transdermal scopolamine). If medical management fails, surgical therapy may be required (see Chapter 7).

Histopathologic examination of temporal bones from patients with Meniere's disease shows distention of the endolymphatic system, with a ballooning of Reissner's membrane (see Figure 4–14). Herniations or ruptures of the wall of the membraneous labyrinth may also be present. The saccule and, to a lesser degree, the utricle may also be distended. Neural structures are usually preserved. The cause of Meniere's disease is unknown but endolymphatic hydrops can be produced by blocking the vestibular aqueduct and destroying the endolymphatic sac, suggesting that a malfunction of this system may play a role in the etiology.

Cogan's syndrome is another idiopathic condition and is characterized by a non-syphilitic interstitial keratitis associated with vertigo and sensorineural hearing loss. Although the cause of this syndrome is not known, treatment with large doses of steroids has been reported as being effective in controlling its manifestations.

Sudden Deafness Syndrome. Sudden idiopathic sensorineural hearing loss can be defined as a hearing loss that occurs over a short period of time (seconds to days), the onset of which is dated exactly. This syndrome is probably much more common than the number of patients seen with this disorder by physicians would suggest, since many patients apparently recover without ever consulting a physician. Those patients who do not recover after a period of time are more likely to consult a physician. The pathophysiology and treatment of sudden sensorineural hearing loss are discussed in Chapter 5.

Presbycusis. It is generally recognized that the incidence of sensorineural hearing loss increases with advancing age. The cause of this hearing loss is unclear. Many older people are assumed to be suffering from presbycusis when, in fact, other etiologic factors are responsible for their hearing loss. Presbycusis is a diagnosis of exclusion and requires that other causes of bilateral progressive sensorineural hearing loss be ruled out before the diagnosis is made.

Presbycusis may be due, in part, to long exposure to environmental noise. Natives of the Sudan, never exposed to the levels of noise intensity encountered in more technologically advanced societies, do not develop presbycusis as rapidly as natives of more industrialized coutries. However, they also do not develop arteriosclerotic heart disease or diverticulosis; therefore it would be overly simplistic to assume that noise was the only etiologic factor.

Schuknecht has classified four types of presbycusis:

1. The most common type is sensory presbycusis, which is characterized histologically by atrophic changes at the basal end of the organ of Corti. Audiometrically, these changes correspond to high tone hearing loss. Speech discrimination remains fairly good despite the degree of sensorineural hearing loss.

2. Neural presbycusis is characterized histologically by a loss of cochlear neurons. Audiometrically, one finds a speech discrimination score that is disproportionately poor when compared with the pure tone thresholds of hearing. Because of the poor speech discrimination, amplification is less beneficial in these patients.

3. Metabolic presbycusis is characterized by atrophy of the stria vascularis. Patients have a flat sensorineural hearing loss and relatively good speech discrimination until later in the disease.

4. Cochlear conductive presbycusis produces a gradually sloping audiogram and speech discrimination more or less in the range one would expect from the level of pure tone threshold. This type of presbycusis has no histologic correlate but is thought to be secondary to stiffening of the basilar membrane.

Miscellaneous. A large number of systemic diseases which are commonly associated with sensorineural hearing loss. Among the most important of these are diabetes mellitus, hypothyroidism (both congenital and acquired), and multiple sclerosis. Most collagen diseases, such as lupus erythematosus, rheumatoid arthritis, periarteritis nodosa, Wegener's granulomatosis, relapsing polychondritis, and temporal arteritis have also been reported as being associated with sensorineural hearing loss.

Treatment

Treatment of sensorineural hearing loss is directed toward prevention and rehabilitation as well as the diagnosis and treatment of other diseases associated with sensorineural hearing loss, some of which may be life threatening.

Prevention

In many instances of inherited sensorineural hearing loss, a family history can be obtained regarding the occurrence of hearing loss. Accurate genetic counseling should be provided to potential parents regarding the possibility of their offspring either having a hearing loss or carrying a recessive gene for hearing loss. In some instances, such as in Tay-Sachs disease, a test for the heterozygous state exists, and the potential carriers, who are almost always Jewish, can be tested and given extremely accurate genetic counseling. In other instances, such as in Refsum's syndrome or chromosomal abnormalities, a prenatal diagnosis can be made by amniocentesis, and if the affected individual is identified, the pregnancy can be terminated.

Very few types of inherited sensorineural hearing loss due to inborn errors of metabolism can be effectively treated with medication although dietary restriction can be helpful in some instances such as in patients with the hyperlipoproteinemias and Refsum's syndrome. There are reports of renal transplantation improving the hearing loss in Alport's syndrome. The use of penicillamine has been reported to improve the hearing loss in patients with retinitis pigmentosa. In this latter case, the penicillamine is thought to bind copper. The incidence of deafness associated with erythroblastosis fetalis can be reduced by the use of RhoGAM to prevent maternal isosensitization. The infant's bilirubin level can be lowered by the use of ultraviolet irradiation, phenobarbital therapy, or exchange transfusions.

It is to be hoped that the incidence of sensorineural hearing loss due to prenatal maternal rubella and postnatal mumps and measles will be reduced by the widespread use of the rubella, rubeola, and mumps vaccines. Further, the development of less ototoxic aminoglycoside antibiotics and better realization by physicians of the risks associated with these drugs, particularly in patients with impaired renal function, can reduce the incidence of this type of sensorineural hearing loss.

In several instances, there are medications that will prevent sensorineural hearing loss. Corticosteroids can reduce the incidence and severity of sensorineural hearing loss in congenital syphilis, and fluorides are thought to stabilize the hearing loss caused by cochlear otosclerosis. It is still uncertain whether calcitonin and similar medications will reverse or limit the hearing loss in Paget's dsease. A large variety of medications, including vasodilators and heparin, have been claimed to be of some value in the treatment of sudden sensorineural hearing loss, but no well-controlled studies are available to support these claims.

The slow sensorineural hearing loss associated with chronic suppurative otitis media and with cholesteatoma can be prevented by appropriate surgical treatment. Surgical repair of round or oval window fistulae and other labyrinthine fistulae can prevent or reverse sensorineural hearing loss. Removal of a poststapedectomy granulomas may restore hearing in those rare instances in which they occur and are diagnosed promptly. Hearing can be preserved in certain cases of acoustic neuroma when they are diagnosed early and are of very small size. Endolymphatic sac procedures may stabilize the hearing in up to two thirds of patients with Meinere's disease.

Perhaps the largest cause of avoidable sensorineural hearing loss is exposure to high-intensity noise. Controlling noise exposure in industry and in the military will prevent a great deal of unnecessary hearing loss from this cause. Public awareness of the risk of noise from such sources as rock bands, motorcycles, and skeet shooting and other sports can be improved by programs that will educate and inform the public.

Rehabilitation

Amplification by the use of a hearing aid is, at present, the major form of rehabilitation available to patients with sensorineural hearing loss. Recent legislation has improved the system of dispensing hearing aids and now a patient must be examined by a physician or sign a waiver prior to obtaining a hearing aid. In the case of an infant with a sensorineural hearing loss it is important that amplification be made available as soon as possible. The fact that brainstem response audiometry now allows objective hearing tests in infants should reduce the unnecessary delays in rehabilitation that were previously encountered. Speech (or lip) reading education can also be of benefit in enabling a patient with a significant sensorineural hearing loss to communicate. Cochlear implants are currently available through established centers in the United States and abroad for profoundly deaf individuals. Although there are a variety of implants presently undergoing clinical trials, the basic apparatus, consisting of an external receiver, transducer, and amplifier, eventually transmits electrical energy to one or more electrodes implanted in the inner ear (Fig. 4–15). The electrode receives electrical signals from the external source either by a percutaneous connector or by electromagnetic induction through intact skin (Fig. 4–16). At

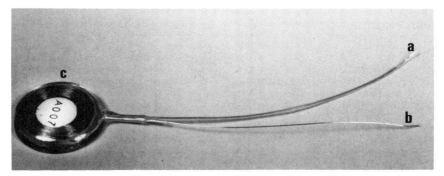

Figure 4–15. Cochlear implant. A = active electrode; B = ground electrode; C = internal induction coil.

the present time, none of the cochlear implant systems is able to restore usable speech discrimination or understanding to the deaf patient. However, despite this limitation, there are many benefits. The speech detection threshold is lowered to a level of 35-to-45-dB hearing level, allowing the patient to hear most medium and loud sounds. Many environmental sounds, such as footsteps, doors slamming, phones ringing, and dogs barking, can be heard, and with training and experience, patients learn to differentiate between these many sounds. By allowing the patient to hear rhythm, pattern, and speech intensity, the implant helps in lip reading. Implant users are able to use the telephone with a simple code, which allows them to carry on limited conversations. Recognition of familiar voices and considerable improvement in their own voice production and quality is possible with the cochlear implant. Many cochlear implant patients notice a decrease in head noise while wearing the stimulator unit. An unmeasurable factor

is the change in quality of life experienced by implant users due to environmental awareness. These individuals feel a greater sense of security, less dependence on others, and more enthusiasm (or less dread) in facing social situations. These observations have been confirmed by close relatives and friends of the implant patients. At the present time, cochlear implants are undergoing clinical trials under Food and Drug Administration regulations governing investigational medical devices. Cochlear implants will most likely play a major role in the future rehabilitation of profoundly deaf individuals.

Treatment of Associated Diseases

It is obvious that even if the hearing is not improved, the patient will benefit from the treatment of the many diseases associated with hearing loss. It has been emphasized

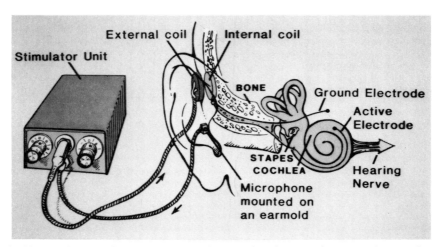

Figure 4–16. Cochlear implant. Artist's rendering of a single electrode induction coil system with external stimulation unit.

that many potentially morbid diseases are associated with sensorineural hearing loss, and the patient's quality and quantity of life may be improved by recognizing and treating these conditions.

BIBLIOGRAPHY

Bergstrom, L., Hemenway, W. G., and Downs, M. A.: A high-risk registry to find congenital deafness. Otolaryngol Clin North Am 4:369–400, 1971.

House, W. F., and Berliner, K. I.: Cochlear implants: progress and perspectives. Ann Otol Rhinol Laryngol 91:11–124, 1982.

Konigsmark, B. S., and Gorlin, R. J.: Genetic and Metabolic Deafness. Philadelphia, W. B. Saunders Co., 1976.

Meyerhoff, W. L.: Medical management of hearing loss. Laryngoscope 88:960–973, 1978.

Meyerhoff, W. L.: Granulomas and other specific diseases of the ear and temporal bone. In Paparella, M. M., and Shumrick, W. B. (eds.): Otolaryngology. Vol. 2. 2nd ed. Philadelphia, W. B. Saunders Co., 1980, pp. 1548–1575.

Meyerhoff, W. L., Liston, S.: Metabolism and hearing loss. In Paparella, M. M., and Shumrick, W. B. (eds.): Otolaryngology. Vol. 2. 2nd ed. Philadelphia, W. B. Saunders Company, 1980, pp. 1829–1845.

Moore, G. R., Robbins, J. P., Seale, D. L., et al: Fluoride and clinical otosclerosis. Arch Otolaryngol 98:327–329, 1973.

Pappas, D. G.: A study of the high-risk registry for sensorineural hearing impairment. Otolaryngol Head Neck Surg 91:41–44, 1983.

Pulec, J. L.: Meniere's disease: etiology, natural history, and results of treatment. Otolaryngol Clin North Am 6:25–40, 1973.

Quick, C. A.: Hearing loss in patients with dialysis and renal transplants. Ann Otol Rhinol Laryngol 85:776–790, 1976.

Schuknecht, H. F.: Pathology of the Ear. Cambridge, Mass., Harvard University Press, 1974.

Spencer, J. T.: Hyperlipoproteinemias in the etiology of inner ear disease. Laryngoscope 83:639–678, 1973.

1) a disease of indeterminant cause; a spontaneous or primary disease

2) A disease generated by an allergy as some forms of eczema; gastro-intestinal disorders

Etiology

1) The science of causes or reasons

2) A branch of medicine that deals with the causes of diseases; also a theory of cause of a particular disease

3) The giving of a cause or reason for anything; also the reason given

Larry G. Duckert
William L. Meyerhoff

5

SUDDEN HEARING LOSS

Any discussion of sudden sensorineural hearing loss should be preceded by a definition of terminology. The hearing loss is always sensorineural, usually unilateral, and accompanied by tinnitus in about 70 per cent of patients. Vertigo is present in 50 per cent of patients. In the past, the term sudden was used to describe a hearing loss that occurred over a period of several seconds up to 5 to 7 days. A more limited and appropriate definition of sudden would include those losses occurring instantaneously or within a matter of hours.

Although sudden sensorineural hearing loss is idiopathic in the majority of cases, a number of etiologic factors have been suggested to be associated with the symptom. When the hearing loss is associated with an identifiable medical problem, treatment should be directed toward correction of this problem. However, the inability of the clinician to identify the exact etiology in most cases results in considerable frustration and empirical treatment. As the pathophysiology of sudden sensorineural hearing loss becomes better understood, treatment can be directed more appropriately, hopefully with more successful results.

In approaching the problem of sudden sensorineural deafness, the suggested pathophysiologic and etiologic theories must first be considered. Recommendations regarding patient evaluation and treatment are based on these theories. The natural history and prognosis of sudden sensorineural hearing loss will also be discussed.

Etiology

A review of the literature concerning the etiology of sudden sensorineural hearing loss confronts the reader with numerous and conflicting theories (Table 5–1). In most cases, the etiology remains speculative, owing to the lack of objective evidence necessary to differentiate the variety of possibilities. Because the cause of the hearing loss is rarely if ever fatal, correlative histopathologic material is scarce. However, despite these limitations, the major known and proposed etiologies of sudden sensorineural hearing loss will be reviewed.

INFECTIOUS THEORY

The hearing loss associated with suppurative labyrinthitis is seldom without predisposing or pre-existing clinical disease, thus making the diagnosis more or less obvious (see Fig. 4–8). The sudden deafness caused by syphilis, however, is frequently less obvious and may be misdiagnosed unless the practitioner maintains a high index of suspicion. The symptoms of syphilitic sensorineural deafness are variable. The disease may present with the symptoms of Meniere's disease, which consist of vertigo, aural fullness, tinnitus, and fluctuating sensorineural hearing loss, or the deafness may be of sudden onset in one ear and rapidly involve the other. Both congenital and acquired forms of syphilis must be considered. The congenital form occurs as a consequence of maternal syphilis and may be expressed either early or later in life. The hearing loss with the early form is usually overshadowed by severe systemic disorders, and for this reason, the latter form is more relevant to this discussion. In this situation, the hearing loss frequently occurs between the eighth and 28th years of life but may be delayed until the fifth decade. Other manifestations of congenital syphilis include interstitial

Table 5–1. ETIOLOGY OF SENSORINEURAL HEARING LOSS

Predisposing Factors	Specific Causes
Diabetes mellitus	Infectious agents
	Bacterial agents
Arteriosclerotic vascular disease (ASVD)	Spirochetal agents
	Fungal agents
Hypertensive heart disease	Viral agents (mumps, adenovirus type III, rubella,
	*Mycoplasma pneumoniae,** influenza, rubeola, herpes
Hyperlipoproteinemia	zoster, Epstein-Barr)
Anxiety	Trauma (temporal bone fracture, perilymphatic leak,
	hemorrhage into the labyrinth)
Allergic diathesis	
	Tumors (petrous apex)
Hypercoagulable states	Toxic agents
	Miscellaneous (Cogan's syndrome, Meniere's syndrome,
	systemic lupus erythematosus, leukemia)

*Arbitrarily grouped with viral agents.

keratitis and dental maldevelopment. Acquired syphilis more commonly produces deafness in the late or tertiary stage, but cases of sudden deafness due to acute meningovascular disease during the secondary stage of syphilis have also been reported.

The histopathology of congenital and acquired syphilis is quite similar. Perivascular mononuclear leukocyte infiltrates are common, as are obliterative endarteritis and temporal bone osteitis, which eventually result in destruction of the membranous labyrinth and associated neurovascular elements.

Viruses are other infectious agents commonly implicated in sudden sensorineural hearing loss. The long list of viruses associated with sudden sensorineural hearing loss includes the viruses of mumps, measles, herpes zoster, chickenpox, and infectious mononucleosis and adenovirus type III. Hearing loss may occur with the clinical syndromes caused by these viruses as well as with subclinical infections diagnosed by serologic techniques.

In 1959, Saunders and Lippy reported several cases of subclinical mumps associated with sudden deafness that were identified using serologic tests. Since then, additional serologic evidence obtained using acute and convalescent viral titers in cases of sudden deafness has incriminated other viral agents, including adenovirus type III and *Mycoplasma pneumoniae* (the latter is not a virus but for convenience will be grouped with the viruses).

Histopathologic data have also supported the concept of virus-related sudden deafness. Pathologic changes present in ears of patients with sudden sensorineural hearing loss of suspected viral etiology include atrophy of the organ of Corti with loss of hair cells and supporting elements. These changes are very similar to those found in labyrinthitis produced by measles and mumps (Fig. 5–1).

Multiple mechanisms for virus-induced hearing loss have been suggested. The viral agents may produce a neuronitis or ganglionitis as a result of viral infiltration of the spiral ganglion and eighth nerve. Viruses may also cause vascular occlusion or result in endolymphatic or perilymphatic labyrinthitis from direct viral invasion. In the case of vascular occlusion, viruses attach to the erythrocytes and cause hemagglutination and endothelial swelling and induce a state of hypercoagulation that compromises the cochlear blood supply.

VASCULAR THEORY

It is widely believed that the majority of cases of sudden hearing loss result from end organ ischemia. Experimental lesions interfering with the blood supply to the inner ear and organ of Corti result in prompt loss of electrophysiologic homeostasis as well as loss of hair cells and ultimately the entire hearing organ. The cochlea is exquisitely sensitive to anoxic changes. Since reduction in oxygen tension within the cochlear duct is associated with a decrease in endocochlear electrical potential and diminished cochlear microphonics, it is not surprising that patients with identifiable vascular and hematologic disease (e.g., macroglobulinemia, sickle cell disease, polycythemia) are subject to sudden deafness. The normally high hematocrit within the stria vascularis

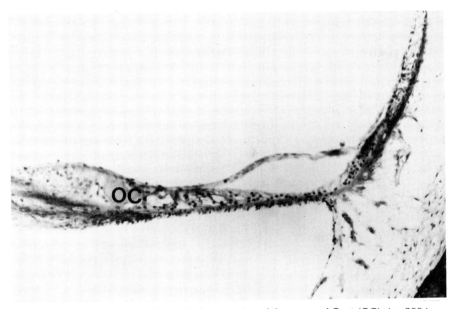

Figure 5–1. Viral labyrinthitis with degeneration of the organ of Corti (OC). (× 300.)

and the slow blood flow lend support to a possible thromboembolic nature of sudden deafness. Sudden sensorineural hearing loss resulting from temporary occlusion, sludging of blood, or vascular spasm are attractive theories in this regard. Other embolic phenomena as well as inner ear hemorrhage have also been associated with sudden deafness (Fig. 5–2).

Evidence of hypercoagulation has been demonstrated in a significant percentage of patients with sudden deafness. These pa-

tients will frequently have other systemic manifestations of hypercoagulability, such as those discussed earlier in the relationship between sudden deafness and virus-induced accelerated coagulation states and vascular damage.

POSSIBLE METABOLIC CAUSES OF SUDDEN DEAFNESS

Sudden deafness may be a local manifestation of a more generalized metabolic im-

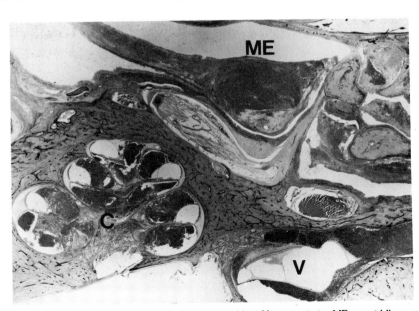

Figure 5–2. Inner ear hemorrhage in leukemia. C = cochlea; V = vestibule; ME = middle ear. (× 10.)

balance. In particular, the high metabolic demands of the stria vascularis within the inner ear make it sensitive to both fluctuation in metabolic rate and availability of certain metabolites. It is therefore not unexpected that certain conditions of metabolic imbalance could have a marked effect on cochlear function. Those conditions that have been associated with sudden deafness include diabetes mellitus and hyperlipoprotinemia. The relationship between sudden sensorineural hearing loss and hypothyroidism and hypoadrenocorticism is less well substantiated.

The association of deficient insulin activity with inner ear dysfunction is well known. Although the mechanisms of hearing loss in diabetes mellitus are not completely understood, microvascular changes and hypoglycemia are two possible means by which labyrinthine function could be adversely affected. The diabetic angiopathy, which is responsible for retinopathy and nephropathy, may also involve the blood vessels of the inner ear, resulting in deafness due to compromised blood flow or hemorrhage. It has also been observed that variations in glucose metabolism can produce marked decreases in cochlear microphonics. This effect has been linked to the very high energy requirement of the inner ear, which is based on oxidative metabolism of carbohydrates. An additional mechanism conceivably responsible for the increased incidence of sudden sensorineural hearing loss in diabetes mellitus could be the primary neuropathy known to occur in that disease.

Histopathologic changes in the inner ears of diabetics include loss of ganglion cells in the spiral canal and vascular changes in the stria vascularis. Some investigators have demonstrated that the microvascular changes seen in the inner ear are identical to the small vessel changes found in diabetic retinopathy and nephropathy, although this is not universally accepted.

Abnormal lipid metabolism with hyperlipidemia frequently is associated with impairment of carbohydrate metabolism. Patients with this disorder may exhibit hyperglycemia or glucose intolerance. Because of the high metabolic demands of the inner ear, these systemic metabolic diseases can be manifested as cochlear malfunctions. Besides the metabolic effect, the atherosclerotic changes secondary to a lipid imbalance may cause ischemic changes within the cochlea, resulting in hearing loss. Hearing loss associated with lipid imbalance or abnormal lipid metabolism is most frequently associated with those types of hyperlipoproteinemia known to cause atherosclerosis. These include type II-A (elevated betalipoprotein and cholesterol), type II-B (elevated betalipoprotein and prebetalipoprotein), and type IV (elevated prebetalipoprotein and triglycerides). It is of interest that the coagulation properties of platelets are also sensitized to epinephrine by hyperlipoproteinemia, which may then contribute to intravascular thrombosis.

RUPTURE THEORY

There is little doubt that sudden sensorineural hearing loss can be caused by ruptures or tears of the delicate membranes within the cochlea. Frequently there will be a history of strenuous physical exertion or activity involving sudden barometric pressure changes (flying and diving) associated with the loss. It has been estimated that 30 per cent of idiopathic losses are secondary to membrane breaks, with approximately one third of these being spontaneous. A perilymph leak at the oval window is usually associated with vestibular symptoms, whereas perilymph at the round window (Fig. 5–3) classically occurs without vertigo or ataxia. Fluctuation in hearing and vertigo may simulate Meniere's disease, and only if the physician maintains a high index of suspicion, will the diagnosis of perilymph fistula be made. The cochlear malfunction is probably a result of mechanical distortion of the cochlear membrane and mixing of intracochlear fluids, resulting in tissue damage and reduction of the endocochlear potential.

MISCELLANEOUS CAUSES OF SUDDEN SENSORINEURAL HEARING LOSS

Many substances have been identified as potentially ototoxic and may cause sudden sensorineural hearing loss. Some of the most common offenders are the aminoglycoside antibiotics (e.g., gentamicin, neomycin, vancomycin, streptomycin, and kanamycin) and diuretics (e.g., furosemide, ethacrynic acid). Hearing loss associated with these agents is frequently severe, irreversible, and associated with vestibular symptoms. Aspirin is probably the most commonly used ototoxic drug and, in sufficient doses, may cause a

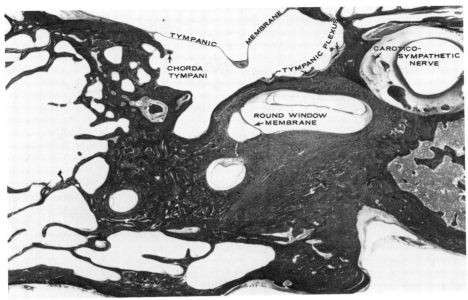

Figure 5–3. Round window membrane. ($\times$ 5.)

hearing loss that fortunately is reversible. Insecticides are among the toxic agents that less commonly produce sudden sensorineural deafness.

Some sensorineural hearing losses are occasionally associated with intracranial neoplasms. Acoustic neuromas present as sudden sensorineural hearing loss in almost 1 per cent of cases (see Fig. 4–12). When abrupt, the hearing loss is probably a result of cochlear ischemia, produced by tumor compression of vascular structures within the internal auditory canal. Meniere's disease may present with sudden sensorineural hearing loss as the initial symptom in approximately 4 per cent of cases, and multiple sclerosis may be implicated in sudden sensorineural hearing loss in 2 per cent of cases. Cogan's syndrome may also present with a sudden sensorineural hearing loss that is bilateral and associated with typical ocular symptomatology.

Diagnosis

Diagnostic evaluation of the patient with sudden sensorineural hearing loss must be sufficiently comprehensive to include all the known diagnostic possibilities already discussed (Table 5–2). Sudden sensorineural hearing loss is an otologic emergency, requiring early evaluation and treatment if a correctable cause is identified. The earlier therapy is begun, the better the prognosis. Complaints of distortion, echoes, and loud-ness intolerance should warrant prompt diagnostic examination.

As with other diagnostic problems, the initial work-up begins with a thorough history and physical examination. The patient should be questioned regarding other medical disorders that could have contributed to the loss. Specifically, information regarding diabetes mellitus, hyperlipidemia, atherosclerotic heart disease, hypertension, and congenital or acquired syphilis should be sought. It should be determined whether these were any potential precipitating events, such as abrupt pressure change, febrile illness, trauma, previous otologic surgery, or drug use. Significant symptoms associated with the hearing loss should also be documented, including time of onset, progression, fluctuation, or the presence of tinnitus or vertigo. A general physical examination with appropriate attention to the affected ear is then completed. Vestibular and neurologic evaluations as well as tuning fork tests are carried out.

A complete battery of audiometric tests are undertaken. If possible, special audiometric tests to aid in determining the site of the lesion are performed. Besides performing routine pure tone threshold audiometry and speech discrimination tests, acoustic reflex and reflex and tone decay tests and tympanometry should be carried out. The vestibular system may also be evaluated with electronystagmography, especially if vertigo accompanies the hearing loss.

Table 5–2. DIAGNOSTIC EVALUATION OF THE PATIENT WITH SUDDEN
SENSORINEURAL HEARING LOSS

History (Otolaryngological and general)

    History of pre-existing medical or surgical problems
    Previous otologic surgery
    Medications
    Family history
    History of precipitating events (e.g., head trauma, changes in barometric pressure)
    History of co-existing symptoms (e.g., tinnitus, vertigo)

Physical Examination

    Otolaryngologic and general with complete neurologic evaluation

Audiology

    Tuning fork tests
    Pure tone air and bone thresholds, speech reception thresholds, speech discrimination, loudness recruitment,
      and stapedius reflex threshold and decay

Vestibular Examination

    Spontaneous and gaze tests
    Positional tests
    Caloric tests

X-ray

    CT of internal auditory canal and cerebellopontine angle
    CT scan with air contrast study of internal auditory canal

Hematologic

    Complete blood count and differential
    Sedimentation rate and platelet count
    Coagulation parameters
      Prothrombin time
      Partial thromboplastin time
      Prothrombin consumption time and clotting time
    Metabolic evaluation
      Fasting blood sugar
      Two-hour glucose tolerance test
      T_3, T_4, cholesterol and triglycerides
      ACTH plasma cortisol stimulation test
    Serologic and immunologic evaluation
      VDRL
      FTA-ABS

If an acoustic neuroma is suspected, computerized tomography (CT) should be performed (see Fig. 4–13). If the results of the CT scan are negative and the diagnosis remains in question, a CT air contrast study of the internal auditory canal is mandatory.

Standard laboratory tests for sudden sensorineural hearing loss should rule out hematologic disorders (e.g., blood dyscrasias, leukemia, sickle cell anemia), metabolic malfunction (e.g., diabetes mellitus, hyperlipidemia, adrenal-pituitary axis abnormalities), hypercoagulation states, and syphilis (Table 5–2). Because of the high percentage of negative venereal disease research laboratory (VDRL) test results in tertiary and late congenital syphilis, fluorescent treponemal antibody absorption (FTA-ABS) or microhemagglutination-treponema pallidum [MHA-TP] testing is required. A single positive FTA-ABS test result, however, should be repeated for confirmation.

Documentation of hypercoagulation may be difficult because of a variety of different laboratory standards. Although the clotting time may provide a simple and quick measure of the clotting process, recent evidence suggests that the prothrombin consumption test may detect hypercoagulation states with more reliability.

With regard to metabolic disorders, a fasting blood sugar and 2-hour postprandial glucose test may be followed by a 5-hour glucose tolerance test if initial data is abnormal. Measurement of triiodothyronine (T_3) and thyroxine (T_4) levels is sufficient to evaluate thyroid function, and the diagnosis of adrenocortical insufficiency may be made using 17-ketosteroid quantification and the adrenocorticotropic hormone (ACTH) plasma cortisol stimulation test. These latter tests are only recommended when a high index of suspicion or an abnormal glucose tolerance test exists. Hyperlipoproteinemia types I to IV may be identified using serum electrophoresis, although abnormal levels of cholesterol and triglyceride may vary according to the patient's age.

Treatment

MEDICAL MANAGEMENT

If a specific etiology can be defined in cases of sudden sensorineural hearing loss, appropriate therapy is directed toward reversing the specific causative process. Unfortunately, in most cases of idiopathic sudden hearing loss, treatment tends to be based on emotional, empirical considerations. In such cases, treatment protocols should be designed based on accepted pathophysiologic standards (Table 5–3). In general, patients with sudden sensorineural hearing loss should be hospitalized and placed at bed rest during evaluation and initiation of therapy.

Luetic deafness, if diagnosed, is treated with 20 million units per day of intravenous aqueous penicillin for 10 days. In addition, prednisone has also been proved effective in reversing the hearing loss and 6090 mg per day administered orally for 1 month has been recommended. The hearing can deteriorate after discontinuing steroids, and a maintenance level may be necessary for life. In this case, alternate day therapy of from 10 to 15 mg of prednisone will help reduce the side effects of long-term treatment. Because multiplication of the *Treponema* organism in the late stages of syphilis may occur only once every 90 days, some authors have recommended that antibiotic treatment be continued over a 3-month period.

Treatment of sudden sensorineural hearing loss related to metabolic and endocrine imbalances is based on correction of the systemic defect. Errors in glucose and lipid metabolism may be compensated for by diet or, when indicated, more aggressive drug therapy. Although hypothyroidism is not a cause of sudden sensorineural hearing loss, reversal of a hypothyroid state may stabilize

or improve progressive sensorineural hearing loss produced by this disorder in approximately 50 per cent of patients. When adrenocortical insufficiency has resulted in inner ear malfunction, treatment with adrenocortical extract may improve the vertigo and tinnitus but will infrequently reverse the hearing loss. Besides acting as a stimulant of corticosteroid production, ACTH has a distinct lipolytic effect, helps to inhibit hypercoagulation, and reduces inflammation. ACTH has also been shown to reduce vasculitis and hypercoagulation as well as inhibit platelet aggregation. The recommended dosage of ACTH is 40 units daily by intramuscular injection.

Other drug therapy in the treatment of sudden sensorineural hearing loss is directed toward improving blood supply, reducing vascular sludging or inflammation, reversing hypercoagulation and thrombus formation, or producing vasodilatation in the inner ear. For reduction of vascular sludging, intravenous infusion of low molecular weight dextran has been suggested. One half liter of 10 per cent solution given over a 4-hour period repeated every 12 hours for 1 week may reduce rouleau formation. It must be pointed out, however, that fatal side effects have been reported with the use of low molecular weight dextran, and there is no proof that it is effective in this situation.

By far the most common agent used to

Table 5–3. MEDICAL TREATMENT PROTOCOL FOR SUDDEN SENSORINEURAL HEARING LOSS

Medication	Proposed Physiologic Action
Heparin (10,000 units by subcutaneous injection every 12 hours)	Anticoagulant, anti-inflammatory, lipolytic, antihistaminic
ACTH (40 units by intramuscular injection daily)	Anti-inflammatory, reduction of platelet adhesiveness, lipolytic, vasodilatation
Low molecular weight dextran (500 units of a 10% solution intravenously over a 4-hour period every 12 hours)	Expansion of plasma volume and increase of cardiac output, increase of vascular profusion and microcirculation, reduction of blood viscosity, reduction in platelet adhesiveness and rouleau formation
Papaverine hydrochloride	Vasodilatation and increase of cochlear blood flow
5% CO_2/95% O_2 (inhalations for 10 minutes four times daily)	Vasodilatation and increase of cochlear blood flow

reverse hypercoagulation is heparin. Heparin exerts its anticoagulant effects specifically in an antiprothrombin action by inhibiting the conversion of prothrombin to thrombin. Heparin may also influence thrombin formation by stimulating lipoprotein lipase formation. It has been demonstrated that there is an inverse relationship between levels of plasma heparin and circulating cholesterol and low-density lipoproteins. The anti-inflammatory and antihistaminic effects of heparin may also prove beneficial. Five to ten thousand units of heparin given by subcutaneous injection every 12 hours has been recommended.

A variety of drugs have been proposed to act as vasodilators in the cochlear vasculature. Among these, orally administered nicotinic acid and intravenous histamine (2.75 gm in 250 cc of 5 per cent dextrose in water) in dosages sufficient to produce a peripheral flush have been most popular. The use of various drugs to induce vasodilatation within the cochlea has recently been challenged by investigators who have found the cochlear vasculature to be only weakly controlled by adrenergic and cholinergic agents whose effects are easily overcome by changes in systemic blood pressure. Nicotinic acid appears to have little, if any, vasodilatory effects on cochlear vasculature and therefore is not recommended.

Other methods of treatment designed to increase cochlear blood flow have been applied with questionable success. Perhaps the most effective agent is carbon dioxide (CO_2). Administration of 5 per cent CO_2 (95 per cent oxygen [O_2]) at a rate of 5 l per minute over 30 minute periods 4 times a day results in vasodilatation of the central nervous system vasculature, including the cochlear vasculature. Other smooth muscle relaxants have been shown in animal experiments to increase cochlear blood flow. Nylidrin hydrochloride and papaverine hydrochloride are two such drugs that have a physiologic basis for use in sudden sensorineural hearing loss. The use of stellate ganglion blocks and various radiopaque dyes to increase cochlear blood flow has not won general acceptance and is of questionable value.

In summary, it would appear that although a number of drug protocols have been proposed and have enjoyed various degrees of popularity, hard evidence based on pathophysiologic observations that these drugs significantly alter the course of idiopathic sudden sensorineural hearing loss is lacking or at least controversial. Despite this, medical therapy continues to be popular in the treatment of idiopathic sudden sensorineural hearing loss. The therapy used by one of the authors (W.L.M.) is outlined in Table 5-3.

SURGICAL MANAGEMENT

Sudden onset sensorineural hearing loss caused by cerebellopontine angle tumors and perilymphatic fistulae requires surgical management. Perilymph leaks occurring through the oval and round windows are surgically accessible for diagnosis and repair. Often the oval or round window areas must be observed over a period of several minutes to identify slow leakage of inner ear fluid. On occasion, however, a leak may be profuse and easily identifiable. Once a leak is identified, closure is achieved using an autograft of fat, vein, or perichondrium. Postoperatively, physical activity is restricted as well as coughing, sneezing, and nose blowing to avoid increases in cerebrospinal fluid pressure. Surgical results are variable and depend to a great extent on the amount of inner ear damage present prior to closure of the fistula.

Natural History and Outcome

It is difficult to assess the results of treatment in cases of sudden sensorineural hearing loss, since the natural course of the disease is frequently unpredictable and variable. Studies describing recovery statistics after specific therapies frequently fail to recognize the significant percentage of patients that will recover spontaneously without treatment. There are also a large number of variables that appear to influence the natural course and prognosis of the disease process.

It was initially believed that those patients who received treatment within the first 10 days after onset of the hearing loss had a better prognosis for recovery. In one series, 75 per cent of patients seen within ten days recovered completely, whereas only 25 per cent of those seen after 10 days recovered to the same degree.

Pre-existing medical problems, including hypertension and diabetes, may adversely affect the chances of hearing recovery. In some studies these diseases were associated with a poor prognosis. However, other investigators have found no correlation between these diseases and prognosis; therefore the relationship remains unclear. Other parameters that generally influence recovery include the patient's age (the elderly do poorly) and the presence of vertigo or a depressed caloric response in the affected ear. Although the severity of the loss does not appear to influence the chance of recovery, patients with low-frequency losses or upward sloping audiometric curves enjoy a more favorable prognosis than those with high-frequency loss or downward sloping curves. Elevated erythrocyte sedimentation rates have also been correlated with a poor prognosis and may be indicative of viral infection.

As stated earlier, the response to therapy is difficult to evaluate, since the disease course is variable and may be influenced by a number of pre-existing conditions. Studies that have attempted to evaluate recovery rates are faced with the problems of random patient selection, divergence of treatment modalities, and absence of uniform methods for reporting results. A recent prospective study on idiopathic sudden sensorineural hearing loss reported that 65 per cent of patients spontaneously recovered hearing to functional levels independent of any type of medical treatment. Another series designed to evaluate the therapeutic methods used for sudden sensorineural hearing loss could find no correlation between types of treatment and hearing recovery, nor did treatment in general seem to influence the outcome. In this latter series, of 50 per cent of patients who exhibited some gain, one third showed slight improvement, one third showed partial recovery, and one third showed complete recovery.

A recently reported treatment protocol consisting of subcutaneous heparin and oral papavarine hydrochloride was used to treat a series of 26 patients with idiopathic sensorineural hearing loss. Treatment was based on the proposed pathophysiology of idiopathic sudden sensorineural hearing loss and proposed pharmacologic properties of the drugs. In this series, 46 per cent of patients experienced complete recovery, 27 per cent experienced partial recovery, and 27 per cent experienced no recovery.

Although there is little agreement regarding therapy and recovery with or without treatment, it is generally agreed that in the absence of treatment, a certain percentage of patients will recover completely, some will improve or remain unchanged, and a small percentage will get worse. In general, somewhere between 25 and 50 per cent of patients will experience little or no recovery, whereas the remaining 50 to 75 per cent will achieve at least partial return of hearing. At this time, little else can be said regarding the efficacy of treatment for idiopathic sudden sensorineural hearing loss. Additional controlled, prospective, double-blind studies are needed to objectively evaluate the various treatment modalities available.

BIBLIOGRAPHY

Byl, F. M.: Sudden hearing loss research clinic. Otolaryngol Clin North Am 11:71–79, 1978.

Fisch, U.: Management of sudden deafness. Otolaryngol Head Neck Surg 91:3–8, 1983.

Goodhill, V.: Labyrinthine membrane rupture in sudden sensorineural hearing loss. Proc R Soc Med 69:565–572, 1976.

Jaffe, B. F.: Hypercoagulation and other causes of sudden hearing loss. Otolaryngol Clin North Am 8:395–403, 1975.

Jaffe, B. F.: Viral causes of sudden inner ear deafness. Otolaryngol Clin North Am 11:63–69, 1978.

Laird, N., and Wilson, W. R.: Predicting recovery from idiopathic sudden hearing loss. Am J Otolaryngol 4:161–164, 1983.

Meyerhoff, W. L.: Management of sudden deafness. Laryngoscope 89:1867–1868, 1979.

Meyerhoff, W. L., and Paparella, M. M.: Medical therapy for sudden deafness In Snow, J. B. (ed.): Controversy in Otolaryngology. Philadelphia, W. B. Saunders Co., 1980, pp. 3–11.

Nadol, J. B., and Wilson, W. R.: Treatment of sudden hearing loss is illogical In Snow, J. B. (ed.): Controversy in Otolaryngology. Philadelphia, W. B. Saunders, 1980, pp. 23–32.

Saunders, W. H.: Symposium on ear disease. Sudden deafness and its several treatments. Laryngoscope 82:1206–1212, 1972.

Saunders, W., and Lippy, W.: Sudden deafness and Bell's Palsy: A common cause. Ann Otol Rhinol Laryngol 68:830–836, 1959.

Schiff, M., and Brown, M.: Hormones and sudden deafness. Laryngoscope 84:1959–1981, 1974.

Schuknecht, H. F., Kimura, R. S., and Naufal, P. M.: The pathology of sudden deafness. Acta Otolaryngol 76:75–97, 1973.

Simmons, F., and Mattox, D.: Natural history of sudden sensorineural hearing loss. Ann Otol Rhinol Laryngol 86:463–480, 1977.

Donald W. Shrewsbury
William L. Meyerhoff

6

TINNITUS

Tinnitus is one of the most common and least understood symptoms encountered by the practicing physician. Inadequate understanding of the etiology combined with a paucity of effective treatments makes this problem a source of frustration for both patient and physician.

Tinnitus aurium was the term used initially to describe the subjective head noise of ringing in the ears. The term is now more comprehensive and defined as an auditory perception of internal origin (noise) rarely heard by others. The nature of the sound varies considerably, but 20 per cent of patients describe it as ringing, buzzing, or steam escaping. Twenty-five per cent of patients will closely compare the sound with a pure tone similar to that heard on an audiometer. The remaining patients describe a variety of sounds (e.g., cricket's chirping). Unlike tinnitus, auditory hallucinations are much more complex sounds, such as voices or music, and suggest a psychiatric disorder or drug intoxication. Tinnitus should also be distinguished from autophony, the hearing of one's own voice or respiratory sounds, which is usually due to a conductive hearing loss or patulous eustachian tube.

The scope of the problem surrounding tinnitus is enormous. Approximately 95 per cent of the normal population has some sort of auditory perception (tinnitus) of less than 20 dB when placed in a perfectly quiet room. Theories regarding the origin of these perceived sounds include the resting discharge of cochlear hair cells, molecular motion of air within the middle ear, and circulating blood in or near the organ of Corti.

Most people are not aware of their slight tinnitus as a result of the masking effect of ambient noise (usually greater than 35 dB). However, despite the masking effect of ambient noise, a number of people do suffer from tinnitus that is severe enough to disturb their existence. Up to 60 per cent of all otologic patients report tinnitus as a sole or attendant complaint. It has been estimated that over 37 million Americans suffer from some degree of this disorder, and 20 per cent of these 37 million people report that the tinnitus significantly affects their daily lifestyle. Tinnitus is frequently charged with interfering with concentration and sleep and, in extreme forms, is cause of serious mental depression and even suicide.

Eighty-five per cent of tinnitus sufferers are 40 years of age or older. Men and women are affected with equal frequency. Fifty per cent of patients describe their tinnitus as being located in one ear, 40 per cent in both ears, and 10 per cent describe it as being located in the head in general. Although only 50 per cent of people presenting with a chief complaint of tinnitus are aware of having any hearing loss, over 90 per cent do, indeed, have an identifiable loss. The hearing loss may be conductive, sensorineural, or mixed.

Most patients can identify a pure tone with or without an associated band of noise as being similar to the noise they experience. The distribution of pitch is fairly even throughout the frequency range of 0 to 9000 Hz, except for an apparent concentration in the 3500- to 5000-cycle range, in which about 35 per cent of the patients describe their central frequency.

Comparing the loudness of the patient's tinnitus with pure tones on a audiometer has resulted in some surprising findings. Despite the considerable distress expressed by patients, 70 per cent of sufferers have tinnitus of 10 dB or less in intensity and only 5 per cent have tinnitus of a magnitude greater than 40 dB. In most patients, it appears that the subjective intensity of the tinnitus is more closely related to anxiety, fatigue, or the quietness of the surroundings rather than the true loudness of the sound itself.

Correlations between tinnitus and types of ear abnormalities are difficult to make. Thus tinnitus associated with conductive hearing loss tends to be lower frequency than that associated with sensorineural hearing loss. In addition, low-frequency tinnitus is usually of greater magnitude than high-frequency tinnitus. The band width of the tinnitus shows no relationship to diagnosis, type of deafness, site of origin, or subjective severity. However, those people who describe their tinnitus as being similar to the sound of steam escaping have the widest band width, those who complain of ringing have the narrowest, and those hearing a buzz have an intermediate width. Although there is no relationship between the subjective severity of tinnitus and its measured volume, there is a correlation between objective band width and volume in that narrow-band tinnitus is usually louder than wide-band tinnitus. Beyond these relationships, few associations can be identified. The central frequency of tinnitus is unrelated to the underlying diagnosis, description, site of origin, or severity. Band width is also unrelated to the central frequency. There is a lack of correlation between the objectively determined loudness of the tinnitus and the diagnosis, type of deafness, site of origin, or amount of audiometrically determined hearing loss.

Researchers who have attempted to understand the etiology of tinnitus have been enormously handicapped by their inability to objectively measure tinnitus directly and by the lack of any suitable animal model. Most explanations regarding the cause of tinnitus are therefore more speculative than objective. Early theories suggested that tinnitus is the result of paresthesia of the auditory nerve; vasospasm secondary to autonomic imbalance; irritation of the tympanic plexus from middle ear inflammation; hypersensitivity of the chorda tympani nerve; intracellular edema of the organ of Corti, bringing the hair cells into steady contact with the tectorial membrane; blood sludging in the inner ear; or the effects of increased tension of the middle ear muscles, compressing the inner ear fluids. Recordings taken from the round window membrane in patients with tinnitus reveal inner ear electrical activity, and metabolic studies in animal models for tinnitus reveal increased activity in the brainstem nuclei.

There are two attractive theories on the origin of tinnitus. One suggests that the cause of tinnitus is related to conditions that increase the excitability of the cochlea, such as irritation from exposure to sound or any steady mechanical pressure that produces a slight but permanent displacement of the tectorial membrane in relation to the hair cells. In the second theory, Hilding has suggested that there might be loss of support for the outer border of the tectorial membrane, allowing it to create tension of the hair cells, thereby causing tinnitus. There is little experimental proof, if any, for either of these two theories, however.

Classification

Many classifications have been proposed for tinnitus. The one proposed by Fowler in 1940 is one of the most useful, since it is applicable to a systematic approach for diagnosis and treatment (Table 6–1). The two major divisions in this classification are vibratory and nonvibratory tinnitus. The first division refers to real sounds, mechanical in origin, airising within or near the ear, whereas nonvibratory tinnitus consists of neural excitation and conduction from anywhere within the auditory system to the auditory cortex without a mechanical basis. Vibratory tinnitus can be subdivided into subjective tinnitus, which is heard only by the patient, and objective tinnitus, which may be heard by interested observers. Nonvibratory tinnitus, which is always subjective and much more common than vibratory tinnitus, is divided into tympanic, petrous, and central, depending upon its proposed origin.

VIBRATORY TINNITUS

As might be expected, vibratory tinnitus is generally better understood, easier to diagnose, and often more readily treatable than nonvibratory tinnitus. There are a variety of

Table 6–1. CLASSIFICATION OF TINNITUS

Vibratory Tinnitus
Subjective
Objective
Nonvibratory Tinnitus
Tympanic
Petrous
Central

Table 6–2. CAUSES OF VIBRATORY TINNITUS

Vascular disorders
    Arteriovenous malformations
    Middle ear inflammation
    Aberrant vessels
    Vascular neoplasms (glomus tympanicum and
       glomus jugulare)
    Dilatations or stenoses of major vessels
Clonic muscular contractions
    Tensor tympani
    Tensor veli palatini
    Stapedius
Patent eustachian tube

pathologic states that cause enough mechanical energy to be heard by others. These are usually vascular, neruomuscular, or those secondary to an abnormally patent eustachian tube. If the noise is loud enough to be heard by others, it is termed objective; otherwise it is termed subjective.

Vascular disorders seem to be the most frequent causative factors of vibratory tinnitus (Table 6–2). Either local or regional vascular changes may result in an increase or change in blood flow with associated turbulance resulting in tinnitus. A fairly common cause is an arteriovenous (A-V) malformation in the posterior cranial fossa. Branches of the occipital artery and transverse sinus are usually involved, although the internal carotid artery and vertebral arteries may also produce audible A-V fistulae. Headaches are frequent when the lesion is intracranial, and up to 50 per cent of patients will have some clinical signs, such as papilledema or a pulsatile mass behind the ear. Tinnitus may be reduced by pressure over the lesion or compression of the feeding artery when possible. Another diagnostic clue in the evaluation of a vascular abnormality is the synchrony between the patient's heartbeat and the tinnitus.

Venous hums, like A-V malformations, are continuous but also have systolic intensification. They become more pronounced during high cardiac output states, such as pregnancy, thyrotoxicosis, or anemia. The Valsalva maneuver decreases the venous hum, whereas turning the head to the opposite side usually increases it. This latter finding is due to ipsilateral contraction of the sternocleidomastoid muscle opening the bore of the internal jugular vein and increasing the turbulence of the jugular blood flow as the vessel bends around the transverse process of the atlas. Acute and chronic middle ear inflammation, aberrant vessels (internal carotid, persistent stapedial artery [see Fig. 6–1], dehiscent jugular bulb), vascular neoplasms, and aneurysmal dilation or partial stenoses of major vessels can also create enough mechanical energy to result in the auditory perception of sound (see Figs. 2–1 and 2–12).

Palatal myoclonus is another entity that gives rise to vibratory tinnitus. This phenomena is the result of clonic muscular contractions of the tensor tympani, stape-

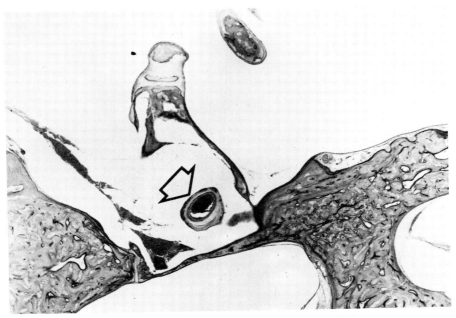

Figure 6–1. Persistent stapedial artery (arrow). (× 20.)

dius, tensor veli palatini, or levator veli palatini muscles. It manifests as a rhythmic audible tinnitus of 10 to 200 clicks per minute, with synchronous movement of the palate and occasionally with lingual or diaphragmatic contractions. Palatal myoclonus is classified neurologically as an extrapyramidal disorder involving the cerebellum. Hemorrhage, thrombosis, embolism, tumor, abscess, multiple sclerosis, syphilis, or malaria may be the underlying cause. Frequently, however, the underlying etiology cannot be identified. The patient may be able to consciously alter the rate of clonic contractions, and tympanic membrane or palatal movement can be recorded on tympanometry or electromyography, respectively.

A patulous eustachian tube may also result in the perception of sound. Normally the eustachian tube is closed. Occasionally it may become abnormally patulous, and the normal nasopharyngeal air turbulence or respiration is transmitted loudly to the middle ear. Autophony, the abnormal awareness of one's own voice, may also be present. This condition is most often seen following a large weight loss, in patients on birth control pills, or during the postpartum period. Otoscopy and tympanometry may reveal tympanic membrane movements associated with respiration. Also, placing the head in a dependent position may cause local venous engorgement and closure of the eustachian tube, with resultant cessation of the auditory symptoms. The injection of inert substances at the eustachian tube orifice in the nasopharynx has been used in the past as a therapeutic modality in the treatment of this type of problem. Unfortunately, a high incidence of middle ear effusion follows this treatment, and it has not gained wide acceptance.

NONVIBRATORY TINNITUS

Nonvibratory tinnitus is less well understood than vibratory tinnitus but is far more common. Various investigators have tried to use the patient's subjective perception of the sound (unilateral, bilateral, or in the center of the head) to distinguish what part of the auditory system is responsible for the origin of the tinnitus. Reed has identified 75 per cent of his tinnitus study group as having a cochlear origin of the sound; 4 per cent, conductive origin; 18 per cent, central nervous system origin; and 3 per cent, vascular origin. Observations that tinnitus persists in a percentage of patients despite destruction of the inner ear or section of the eight cranial nerve lends credence to the concept of central tinnitus.

Some known causes of central tinnitus are space-occupying lesions, inflammation, and vascular abnormalities (Table 6–3). Frequently, however, none of these conditions is present and the patient still suffers from central tinnitus. The "gate theory" of Melzack and Wall suggests that efferent pathways control the presynaptic mechanisms, which in turn control the ease with which cochlear information can enter the brainstem. Alteration of this system may allow central input out of proportion to peripheral input.

Lempert advocated typanosympathectomy to destroy what he believed were connections between the middle ear autonomic nervous system and the cochlea. These autonomic connections were also proposed to be the cause of tinnitus associated with Costen's syndrome (temporomandibular joint dysfunction and occasional tinnitus). This theory is not well regarded by many of today's otologists, and tympanosympathectomy has been abandoned as a cure for tinnitus.

Diagnosis

HISTORY

Evaluation of the tinnitus starts with a thorough history. An attempt should be made to ascertain the age of onset, mode of progression, family history, and association with other audiovestibular symptoms (hearing loss, aural fullness, and vertigo). General information should be gathered about the location (general, unilateral, bilateral); pitch (high, low); relative complexity (single sound, multiple sounds); pattern (steady, pulsatile, clicking); apparent intensity; level of aggravation; effect of ambient noise (increasing intensity, decreasing intensity); and duration (continuous intermittent) of the tinnitus. While obtaining these data, it should be recognized that, as noted before, the patient's subjective descriptions often have no correlation to the actual acoustic properties, the underlying cause of the tinnitus, or the site of the lesion. However, one can often derive considerable appreciation for the true nature of the patient's problem in such a detailed history. Also, in the future, with

Table 6–3. CAUSES OF NONVIBRATORY TINNITUS

Presbycusis
Trauma
    Head trauma
    Acoustic trauma
Medication
Conductive hearing loss
Tumor
    Eighth cranial nerve
    Temporal lobe
Meniere's disease
Metabolic disorder
    Diabetes mellitus
    Hypothyroidism
Labyrinthitis
    Allergic
    Viral
    Bacterial
    Spirochetal
Bell's palsy
Otosclerosis
Circulatory disturbance
    Hypertension
    Arteriosclerotic vascular disease

better understanding of the pathophysiology of tinnitus, relationships with elements of the history may become apparent. Lastly, this history serves as a starting point for the classification of the tinnitus.

Additional otologic history should be obtained, such as information regarding aural discharge, head trauma, noise exposure, or exposure to ototoxic drugs. Inquiries about general medical conditions should be made. Special attention should be directed to neurologic symptoms; cardiovascular abnormalities, such as hypertension and arteriosclerosis; metabolic disorders, such as hypothyroidism; or hematologic disorders, such as anemia or leukemia. A history of specific drug ingestion should be obtained. These drugs include alcohol, salicylates, caffeine, tobacco, antimicrobial agents (e.g., aminoglycosides), and thyroid medication. A Minnesota Multiphasic Personality Inventory and general psychologic evaluation have prognostic as well as diagnostic value. Since the degree to which patients suffer from tinnitus is not necessarily related to the intensity of the tinnitus, this latter examination should be considered only for particularly distraught patients. As discussed under treatment, these patients may benefit from psychologic consultation and biofeedback.

PHYSICAL EXAMINATION

The patient should have a complete neurologic and head and neck examination, with special emphasis on auscultation of the mastoid tip, ear, eye, skull, and neck. Otoscopic inspection should be combined with tuning fork examination and pneumatic otoscopy. Vital signs will reveal signs of hypertensive and orthostatic cardiovascular problems.

Particular attention should be directed to those parts of the history and physical examination that suggest a mechanical basis for the tinnitus. A new technique, phonocephalography, which uses a stethoscope for sound pickup and a phonocardiographic apparatus for sound amplification, may be necessary to locate the source of the patient's vibratory tinnitus. Angiography confirms the presence and location of vascular lesions and should be performed in patients with pulsatile vibratory tinnitus. Tympanometry helps to identify subtle movements of the tympanic membrane due to changes in nasopharyngeal pressure that result from respiratory movements transmitted through a patulous eustachian tube. It will also help in the identification of myoclonus of the stapedial muscle, tensor tympani, and muscles of the palate. Electromyography will confirm the presence of myoclonus of the palatal muscles. Once identified, the cause of palatal myoclonus should be sought.

As mentioned earlier, there is poor correlation between the subjective properties of the nonvibratory variety of tinnitus and the objective findings. For this reason, audiometry plays a substantial role in the evaluation of the patient suffering from nonvibratory tinnitus. A detailed examination begins with the measurement of pure tone threshold and includes Békésy audiometry, if available, to ensure that hearing is sampled in all possible ranges. Attempts to match tinnitus to pure tone sound by Békésy audiometry may produce reasonable approximation by narrow band noise in the same frequency range (see Chapter 8). Patients with high-frequency hearing loss and tinnitus are frequently unaware of any hearing problem. This is understandable in view of the fact that hearing loss is out of the speech frequencies.

The discovery of a hearing loss warrants a full evaluation for determination of the site of lesion and cause. The examination proceeds at this point as if the hearing loss were the chief complaint. Speech discrimination should be tested with and without background noise. Tone decay tests should be performed as well as alternate binaural loudness balance, typanometry (stapedial reflex and reflex decay, tympanic membrane compliance), short increment sensitivity index, and, if indicated, brainstem response audiometry.

Further investigation into the known causes of tinnitus should be performed as indicated by the findings on the history, physical examination, and audiometric profile. Electronystagmography will quantify abnormalities of the vestibular system and plain x-rays, tomograms, and computed tomography (with or without intrathecal air contrast) will identify cerebellopontine angle lesions. Laboratory data, such as tests for syphilis, hemoglobin, and thyroxine levels and glucose tolerance tests, are useful indicators of systemic disease that cause tinnitus. Unilateral tinnitus, in the absence of physical findings, should be evaluated in a fashion similar to unilateral sensorineural hearing loss (see Chapter 4).

Attempts to objectively match the tinnitus to pure tones or more complex sounds is sometimes useful. The nature of the tinnitus is often such that matching is quite difficult due to the narrow band or complex sounds of the tinnitus itself. Basic audiometers provide tones at octave or half octave intervals and at least one form of noise. More complex models, which are capable of producing several noises (white, complex or sawtooth, speech spectrum, and/or narrow band) are more useful in tinnitus masking. Recently, complex music synthesizers have been used to considerably enlarge the spectrum of noise available for tinnitus matching. If the tinnitus is equal in both ears, the technique used for matching is one of monaural loudness balance, in which the tinnitus alone is compared with tinnitus plus matching noise both for loudness and special content. An easier approach is to make the criteria for description less stringent by simply seeking a noise that will mask the tinnitus. The task becomes one of obtaining increasingly fewer approximations of the minimal spectrum necessary to just barely mask the tinnitus. Originally thought of as a research technique with limited practical application, tinnitus matching and masking has assumed an important role in the therapy of tinnitus with the advent of the tinnitus masker.

Treatment

In general, the treatment of tinnitus has been disappointing. The great majority of patients suffer from nonvibratory tinnitus of obscure etiology, which responds poorly to traditional therapies. Despite this, several important points should be understood by the physician. First, a very small percentage (less than 25 per cent) of patients suffering from tinnitus have vibratory tinnitus or nonvibratory tinnitus of an identifiable etiology, such as otosclerosis. It is incumbent upon the physician to identify individuals with the vibratory type and treat the underlying disease process. Secondly, in the past few years there have been some very exciting therapeutic developments, such as the tinnitus masker and biofeedback therapy. Neither of these modalities is the final answer for all patients with nonvibratory tinnitus, although they can provide relief for some tinnitus sufferers. When no treatable cause is uncovered, tinnitus patients are often comforted by simple reassurance and understanding on the part of their physician. Careful explanation that the ringing in their ears is not caused by a brain tumor, infection, or impending stroke is often sufficient therapy.

Surgery has a small but very important role in the treatment of tinnitus. Most causes of vibratory tinnitus are amenable to surgery. The tinnitus of cerebellopontine angle lesions, temporal lobe neoplasm, and conductive hearing loss can frequently be improved or relieved by surgery, although the results are inconsistent and unpredictable.

Removal of an intracranial A-V malformation or one in the vicinity of the ear will relieve the tinnitus as well as any associated high-output heart failure. In the case of venous hum, some patients are so bothered by the tinnitus that jugular vein ligation may be offered as a treatment. Section of the levator veli palatini has been described as a treatment for some forms of palatal myoclonus; however, because of inconsistent and unpredictable results, this operation has failed to gain widespread support among otolaryngologists. In the case of myoclonus of the stapedial muscle or tensor tympani muscle, section of the offending muscle is curative. In those patients afflicted with otosclerosis, up to 75 per cent will experience at least some relief of their tinnitus following stapedectomy. The placement of tympanostomy tubes for patients suffering from middle ear effusion is often helpful in relieving associated tinnitus; however, in the absence of middle ear abnormalities, there is no rationale for their routine use as a treatment for tinnitus.

Numerous operations have been described for the relief of Meniere's disease. Procedures on the endolymphatic sac, ultrasound therapy of the inner ear, cryotherapy to the horizontal semicircular canal, sodium chloride crystals placed at the round window membrane, stellate ganglion sympathectomy, and intermittent repetitive sacculotomy have all provided relief of tinnitus in 30 to 50 per cent of patients with endolymphatic hydrops as the underlying etiology. Labyrinthectomy or eighth cranial nerve section or both have been advocated for those who describe their tinnitus as totally disabling. Unfortunately, these operations sacrifice hearing and relieve tinnitus only in approximately 75 per cent of patients.

As mentioned earlier, one of the older theories regarding the etiology of tinnitus concerns autonomic imbalance. Lempert was the first to propose sectioning the autonomic nerves of the middle ear as a treatment for tinnitus. Although surgical destruction of the chorda tympani and tympanic plexus has largely been discarded as a treatment for tinnitus, otologists in the Soviet Union have described a chemical tympanosympathectomy using lidocaine, procaine, or alcohol ethylmorphine hydrochloride delivered as a subcutaneous injection into the tympanic promontory. They report that almost 50 per cent of patients so treated experienced relief of tinnitus. This form of therapy is not widely practiced in Western countries.

Those who believe that tinnitus is the result of inner ear vasospasm have proposed a temporary chemical or permanent surgical sympathectomy. Golding-Wood reported that 23 per cent of 30 patients with non-Meniere's tinnitus experienced improvement of the tinnitus following sympathectomy. Percutaneous sympathetic blocks were performed with local anesthetics as a therapeutic trial. Occasionally, after several temporary blocks, relief was permanent. In those cases in which the tinnitus recurred, surgical sympathectomy was performed.

Although a number of medications have been proposed at one time or another for the relief of tinnitus, most are based on speculative theories as to the etiology of tinnitus and have not been consistently efficacious over time.

Older nostrums were aimed at increasing the blood flow to the cochlea and central nervous system based on the theory that end-organ ischemia was the cause of tinnitus. To this end, adrenergics, adrenergic-blocking agents, antiadrenergics, anticholinesterase agents, cholinolytics, smooth muscle relaxants, plasma polypeptides, vitamins, and many other drugs have been tried. From animal research, Snow and Suga have concluded that papaverine hydrochloride is the drug of choice to increase cochlear blood flow; however, its efficacy in the treatment of tinnitus is controversial. Vitamins such as vitamin A, vitamin C, nicotinic acid, and vitamin B_{12} have been advocated primarily because of their proposed beneficial effects on the nervous and vascular system. Antihistamines and decongestants have been used when eustachian tube dysfunction is believed to play a role. Tranquilizers have been suggested by some to be of use in reducing the anxiety associated with tinnitus.

One form of therapy that is presently receiving much attention is the use of oral and intravenous anticonvulsant agents. This is based on the theory that some varieties of tinnitus are "epileptiform" in nature. These drugs are believed to stabilize nervous tissue membranes and in some way reduce the tinnitus at its source or within the central level where it is perceived. Melding and associates, who have pioneered this treatment, advocate it for those who have tinnitus with sensorineural hearing loss due to damage in the organ of Corti. These investigators believe that deafferentation of the auditory pathway leads to neuronal hyperactivity causing tinnitus. As they describe the treatment regimen, lidocaine is initially used as a therapeutic test in tinnitus patients. Intravenous lidocaine stabilizes neuronal hyperactivity. Regardless of the mechanism, the authors have found that the majority of patients with nonvibratory tinnitus have partial or complete relief lasting several minutes to several days after the slow intravenous administration of 2 mg per kg of lidocaine. A large percentage of the patients that respond to the intravenous lidocaine will also respond to oral carbamazepine (Tegretol) and a smaller percentage will respond to diphenylhydantoin (Dilantin). Patients that fail to respond to lidocaine receive little if any benefit from carbamazepine.

In addition to their use in idiopathic nonvibratory tinnitus, there have also been reports of Tegretol or Dilantin being successful in treating the tinnitus of palatal myoclonus. Any physician prescribing Tegretol should be aware of the side effect of refractory

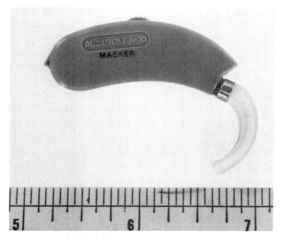

Figure 6–2. A tinnitus masker (scale in inches).

aplastic anemia, which occurs occasionally with its prolonged use. One should also be aware that this form of therapy for tinnitus is new, and long-term follow-up is currently lacking. Many patients, however, continue to be significantly distraught in spite of a complete medical evaluation, reassurance, and trial of medical therapy.

The fact that tinnitus can be masked has been known for many years, but it is only recently that masking has been systematically employed in the treatment of tinnitus patients. Several modalities are employed to achieve tinnitus masking. All of them should be used only after a thorough medical evaluation has been performed and the range and volume of the patient's tinnitus has been carefully plotted, using comparison with tones from an audiometer. First, an attempt is made to characterize the tinnitus within the narrowest limits possible. Patients with a high-frequency hearing loss corresponding to the narrow band of tinnitus perceived often benefit from a hearing aid that selectively amplifies high-frequency sounds.

Recently, a new appliance has been developed called a tinnitus masker. In appearance, it is quite similar to a behind-the-ear or in-the-ear hearing aid (Fig. 6–2). It provides a band of noise starting above the speech frequencies and extending to as high a frequency as possible with an adjustable volume of 40-dB to 85-dB SPL (sound pressure level). It may be used ipsilaterally or contralaterally, although contralateral use is far less effective. The band of noise pro-

duced by the tinnitus masker masks the patients' tinnitus and substitutes a sound that the patients often find less annoying than the sound of their own tinnitus. Being an external noise, it is more easily ignored or suppressed by patients. Eighty per cent of carefully selected patients report complete relief of their tinnitus, whereas the rest seem to obtain some degree of partial relief. Interestingly, many patients report residual inhibition of their tinnitus after they stop using their ipsilateral tinnitus maskers. This inhibition lasts from a fraction of a minute to up to 2 days and is related somewhat to the duration the masker was used continuously before it was removed. Contralateral masking does not elicit this interesting phenomenon.

The tinnitus masker may be combined with an amplifier in the same device. As might be expected, profoundly deaf people obtain little benefit from the masker, and there are also obvious limitations in attempting to mask tinnitus in the speech reception frequencies.

The last modality for the masking of tinnitus is the technique of "de-tuning" an FM radio at bedtime in an effort to mask the tinnitus with radio static. Patients can select as wide a noise band as they wish. This method of relief is particularly suited to those patients who experience discomfort only at night or during times of quiet concentration.

In many cases the disability attributed to tinnitus is more a reflection of the patient's subjective response to tinnitus than to the real intensity of the sound. This theory is supported by the finding that the patient's subjective assessment of the loudness of his tinnitus is unrelated to the real intensity as identified by tinnitus matching. Although many patients complaining of tinnitus have made some emotional adjustment to it, there are a large group of patients whose tinnitus is extremely aggravating and causes significant difficulty in their daily lives. Many of these people are presently using or have tried modalities such as tranquilizers, hypnosis, psychotherapy, or acupuncture. These people may be candidates for biofeedback. Biofeedback is a well-established technique for modifying stress and pain reactions to physical problems. It is an attempt to exert conscious control over areas of the body previously thought to be out of the control of the conscious mind. In a serious of sessions, the patient learns relaxation exercises and ways of relieving stress-related muscle tension or spasm. The patient is not only taught to relax but also encouraged to relate the state of relaxation to the stress of day-to-day living experiences. Ultimately, the patient learns to control his or her level of relaxation, thus reducing stress and its symptoms, one of which is tinnitus.

Considering that patients selected for biofeedback therapy have usually been refractory to other forms of tinnitus therapy, results have definitely been encouraging. A small percentage of patients report complete disappearance of tinnitus, whereas the majority obtain some degree of relief. A small number will experience return of their discomfort to the previous level, but in most cases, the success of this therapy is documented by decreased reliance on other forms of therapy such as tranquilizers. It should be noted that few otologists are trained to supervise this therapy, and psychologists familiar with the technique should design the program to objectively evaluate pre- and post-therapy effects.

One of the more experimental forms of tinnitus therapy involves galvanic stimulation of the cochlea. Stimulation of the cochlea during auditory rehabilitation of the profoundly deaf has occasionally relieved tinnitus for variable periods of time. Further studies have demonstrated that tinnitus suppression occurred during positive pulse stimulation without affecting acoustical perception or hearing. Up to 50 per cent of patients having undergone cochlear implantation report a significant decrease in their preoperative tinnitus. More investigation is needed to establish electrical stimulation of the cochlea as a practical therapy.

BIBLIOGRAPHY

Adlingron, P., and Warrick, J.: Stellate ganglion block in the management of tinnitus. J Laryngol Otol 85:159–168, 1971.

Cazals, Y., Negrevergne, M., and Aran, J. M.: Electrical stimulation of the cochlea in man: hearing induction and tinnitus suppression. J Am Audiol Soc 3:209–213, 1978.

Englesson, S., Larsson, S., Lindquist, N. C., et al: Accumulation of 14C-lidocaine in the inner ear. Preliminary clinical experience utilizing intravenous lidocaine in the treatment of severe tinnitus. Acta Otolaryngol (Stockh) 82:297–300, 1976.

Fowler, E. P.: Intravenous procaine in the treatment of Meniere's disease. Ann Otol Rhinol Laryngol 62:1186–1200, 1953.

Fowler, E. P.: Head noises. Arch Otolaryngol 32:903–914, 1940.

Golding-Wood, P. H.: The role of sympathectomy in the treatment of Meniere's disease. J Laryngol Otol 83:941–947, 1969.

Graham, J. T., and Newby, H. A.: Acoustical characteristics of tinnitus. Arch Otolaryngol 75:82–87, 1962.

Hilding, A. C.: Studies on the otic labyrinth. The possible relation of the insertion of the tectorial membrane to acoustic trauma, nerve deafness, and tinnitus. Ann Otol Rhinol Laryngol 62:470–476, 1953.

House, J. W.: Treatment of severe tinnitus with biofeedback training. Laryngoscope 88:406–412, 1978.

Lemport, J.: Tympanosympathectomy: Surgical technic for relief of tinnitus aurium. Arch Otolaryng 43:199–212, 1946.

Melding, P. S., Goodey, R. J., and Thorne, P. R.: The use of intravenous lidocaine in the diagnosis and treatment of tinnitus. J Laryngol Otol 92:115–121, 1978.

Melzack, R., and Wall, P. D.: Pain mechanisms: A new theory. Science 150:971–979, 1965.

Meyerhoff, W. L., and Cooper, J. C.: Tinnitus. In Paparella, M. M., and Shumrick, D. A. (eds.): Otolaryngology. Vol 2. 2nd ed. Philadelphia, W.B. Saunders Co., 1980, pp. 1861–1870.

Reed, G. F.: An audiometric study of two hundred cases of subjective tinnitus. Arch Otolaryngol 71:95–104, 1960.

Snow, J. B., and Suga, F.: Control of the microcirculation of the inner ear. Otolaryngol Clin North Am 8:455–466, 1975.

Vernon, J., and Schleuning, A.: Tinnitus: A new management. Laryngoscope 88:413–419, 1978.

Hubert Vermeersch
William L. Meyerhoff
René Boothby

7

VERTIGO

There is a close anatomic relationship between the peripheral auditory system and the peripheral vestibular system, and therefore, disorders of the latter frequently accompany hearing loss. The resultant disturbance in balance may take one of several forms and may, indeed, be the most incapacitating symptom. Since terminology on this subject is rather confusing, the discussion of vertigo will be preceded by a definition of terms.

Dizziness and *giddiness* are general nonspecific terms referring to any altered orientation in space. *Vertigo* is a specific type of dizziness, which is defined as an illusion or hallucination of rotatory motion. Whether the illusion is that of a person spinning in a stationary environment or the environment spinning around the person is unimportant in diagnosing the underlying cause. Also, the direction of the spinning sensation appears to be of little diagnostic import. Some clinicians extend the definition of vertigo to include any hallucination of motion, spinning or not, and it is well documented that such nonrotatory sensations are frequently vestibular in origin.

Unsteadiness and *lightheadedness* often serve as a prodrome or residual of true vertigo or they may exist as separate entities unrelated to vestibular disease. *Ataxia* (the failure of muscle coordination) and *gait disturbance* may also be symptoms of vestibular disease and occasionally occur in patients with acoustic neuroma, in which true vertigo is unusual owing to the slow growth of the tumor. *Syncope, fainting,* and actual *loss of consciousness,* however, are not forms of dizziness and have different diagnostic implications, usually cardiovascular.

In order to adequately evaluate a patient who is complaining of spacial disorientation, the physician must first obtain a description of the patient's sensations during the dizzy spells. The history remains the most important step in the evaluation of this problem. To avoid possible oversight, the investigator should prepare a question list that can be completed by the patient. An example of a rather complete register is given in Table 7–1. Appropriate history, diagnostic tests, and laboratory evaluation that should accompany this questionnaire are outlined in Table 7–2. Their purpose will be better understood after discussion of the normal maintenance of equilibrium in man.

Anatomy and Physiology

Peripheral and central vestibular pathways play major roles in the balance regulatory system, but normal appreciation of spacial orientation also requires integration of ocular and proprioceptive centers. This integration takes place in the reticular formation and the cerebellum. These latter centers must be kept in mind when dealing with a patient with dysequilibrium.

The vestibular labyrinth consists of three semicircular canals (anterior or superior, horizontal or lateral, and inferior or posterior), the utricle, and the saccule (Fig. 7–1). It lies within the temporal bone, and its inner membranous portion is surrounded by perilymph.

The three semicircular canals, which lie at 90-degree angles to each other, are not gravity-dependent organs but rather respond only to angular acceleration. The ampullae, saccular dilatations of the semicircular canals that house the cristae (sensory epithelium), are located anteriorly on the horizontal and superior canals and posteriorly on the posterior canal. The most peripheral sensory component of the vestibular system is the hair cell (Type I and Type II) (Fig. 7–2).

Table 7–1. VESTIBULAR EVALUATION

Name _____ Age _____ Date _____

Address _____ City _____ State _____

	Yes	No	
1. Is your dizziness			Give date that your dizziness started:
Lightheadedness	_____	_____	
Swimming sensation	_____	_____	
Wooziness	_____	_____	_____
Faintness	_____	_____	
Blacking out (unconsciousness)	_____	_____	Frequency of attacks:
Turning or spinning	_____	_____	
Side-to-side movement	_____	_____	
Up-and-down movement	_____	_____	_____
Falling sensation	_____	_____	
2. Is your dizziness			
Sudden in onset	_____	_____	
Gradual in onset	_____	_____	
Constant	_____	_____	
In attacks that last			
Seconds	_____	_____	
Minutes	_____	_____	
Hours	_____	_____	
Days	_____	_____	
3. Do you have a warning prior to an attack?	_____	_____	
4. Is your dizziness accompanied by			
Nausea	_____	_____	
Vomiting	_____	_____	
Rapid heart beat	_____	_____	
Sweating	_____	_____	
5. Is your dizziness related to meals?	_____	_____	

	Yes	No	Yes	No
			Is it made worse by	
6. Is it brought on by				
Walking	_____	_____	_____	_____
Sitting up	_____	_____	_____	_____
Lying down	_____	_____	_____	_____
Standing	_____	_____	_____	_____
Arising from lying down	_____	_____	_____	_____
Turning	_____	_____	_____	_____
Walking in dark	_____	_____	_____	_____
7. Are you completely free of dizziness between attacks?	_____	_____		
8. Do you know of anything that will				
Stop your dizziness or make it better	_____	_____		
Make your dizziness worse	_____	_____		

Table 7–1. VESTIBULAR EVALUATION (*Continued*)

9. Do you suspect a cause for your dizziness? ———— ———— If yes, what?

————————

10. Do you have hearing loss in your
      Right ear ———— ————
      Left ear ———— ————

11. Do you have ringing in your ears?
      Right ear ———— ————
      Left ear ———— ————

12. Do you feel pressure in your ears?
      Right ear ———— ————
      Left ear ———— ————

13. Do you have discharge from your ears?
      Right ear ———— ————
      Left ear ———— ————

14. Do you have double or blurry vision? ———— ————

15. Were you exposed to any irritating fumes, paints, etc., at the onset
      of your dizziness? ———— ————

16. Do you have any allergies? ———— ————
      To what? ————————————————————

17. Have you ever injured your head? ———— ————
      Were you unconscious? ———— ————

18. Had you been taking any medications regularly before your
      dizziness started? ———— ————

      What? ————————————————————

19. Do you drink alcohol? ———— ————

      How much? ————————————————————

20. Have you ever smoked or do you now smoke? ———— ————
      How much? ————————————————————
      How long? ————————————————————

21. Have you ever been told you had either high or low blood
      pressure? ———— ————
      Which? High ———— Low ————

Table 7–2. DIAGNOSTIC PROTOCOL FOR VERTIGO

History

Otolaryngologic History
   Establish the nature of dizziness as well as frequency, duration, and precipitating factors
   Establish the presence of associated symptoms: hearing loss, otorrhea, head trauma, noise exposure, tinnitus, otalgia, aural fullness, diplacusis, recruitment, Tullio's phenomenon, nausea, and vomiting
Complete General History
   Hypothyroidism, adrenocortical insufficiency, blood dyscrasias, visual disturbance, arteriosclerotic vascular disease, diabetes mellitus, collagenoses, allergy, renal disease, syphilis, and medications

Physical Examination

Otolaryngologic
   External ear and tympanic membrane, cranial nerves, spontaneous nystagmus, fistula test, Romberg test, past pointing, Hennebert's sign, dysdiadochokinesia
General
   Vascular and systemic diseases as suggested by history
Neurologic
   Cerebellar signs, seizures, multiple sclerosis

Audiologic Test Battery

   Tuning fork tests (e.g., Rinne, Weber)
   Pure tone audiometry
   Speech reception threshold
   Tone decay tests
   Loudness recruitment tests (short increment sensitivity index [SISI] test, alternate binaural loudness balance [ABLB] test)
   Békésy and comfortable loudness Békésy tests
   Binaural pitch masking
   Impedance audiometry and stapedial reflex testing (including stapedial reflex decay)
   Auditory brainstem response (ABR)

Electronystagmography

   Spontaneous nystagmus
   Provoked nystagmus
      Positional tests
      Caloric tests (air caloric and water caloric)
      Eye-tracking tests
      Optokinetic tests (Bárány)
      Calibration
      Rotatory testing
      Posturography

Radiology

   Skull
   Mastoid and internal auditory canals
   Polytomography of the internal ear
   Clivogram (posterior fossa myelogram) and pneumencephalography
   Computed tomography
   Nuclear magnetic resonance
   Angiography
   Cervical spine

General Examinations

   Cardiovascular (electrocardiogram [EKG])
   Hematology (white blood count [WBC], hemoglobin [HGB], sedimentation rate, electrolytes, lipid analysis, coagulation studies)
   Endocrine (ACTH, thyroid function tests, diabetes)
   Serologic and immunologic evaluation (FTA-ABS, lupus erythematosus cell preparations)
   Lumbar puncture (syphilis, multiple sclerosis, culture for meningitis, cell block)
   Viral studies (stool, CSF, serum)

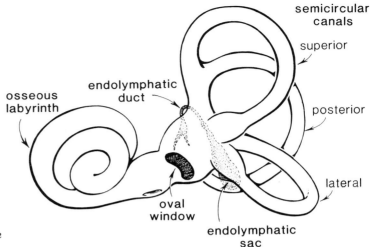

Figure 7–1. Schematic drawing of the vestibular labyrinth.

These hair cells, their supporting cells, and the glycoproteins secreted by the supporting cells make up the crista ampullaris and cupula, respectively (Figs. 7–3 and 7–4). Stereocilia and a kinocilium project from the hair cells into the cupula and are arranged asymmetrically so that the kinocilium lies on the circumference and the stereocilia are located on the remaining portion of the projecting surface of the hair cell. The end-organs of the normal vestibular system are bilateral and physiologically symmetric at rest, with constant and equal discharge coming from both sides. The sensation of vertigo is experienced when these two sides become unequal in their discharge rate. The physiology of the hair cells is such that when the cupula is deflected by inertia of endolymph during angular acceleration, the stereocilia are also deflected. When the stereocilia are bent toward the kinocilium, the cell becomes hyperexcitable, and when the stereocilia are bent away from the kinocilium, the opposite occurs. These hair cells are further arranged within each ampulla so that when endolymph motion causes the cupula to be deflected toward the utricle (utriculopetal), there is afferent neural excitation from the horizontal canal and neural inhibition in the posterior and superior semicircular canals. When angular acceleration results in endolymph motion causing deflection of the cupula away from the utricle (utriculofugal), the opposite occurs.

The hair cells in the utricle and saccule are located in the maculae. The macula utriculi lies in a horizontal plane and the macula sacculi lies in a vertical plane. This specialized patch of membrane is composed of a mucopolysaccharide gel, containing calcareous deposits (otoliths or otoconia) (Fig. 7–5). It is the weight of the otoconia that makes the utricle and saccule gravity-dependent

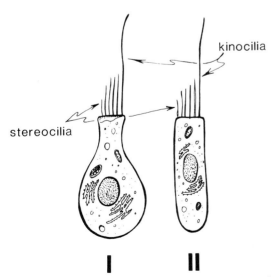

Figure 7–2. Schematic drawing of vestibular hair cells (Type I and Type II).

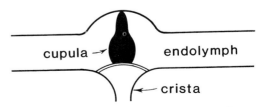

Figure 7–3. Schematic drawing of a semicircular canal ampulla.

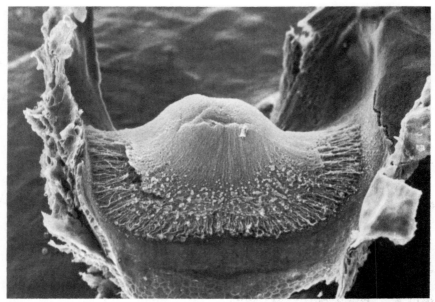

Figure 7–4. Lateral crista of mouse with cupula in place. (× 436.) (Courtesy of Charles G. Wright.)

organs. The movement of these deposits causes a bending of the cilia, which are responsible for initiating electrical impulses transmitted to the brainstem by branches of the vestibular nerves.

Innervation of the vestibular hair cells is both efferent and afferent. Since the exact function and anatomy of the efferent vestibular neural system is not totally understood, discussion will be limited to the afferent system. The information gained by the peripheral vestibular system is transmitted to the central vestibular system by the superior and inferior divisions of the vestibular portion of cranial nerve VIII. The primary afferent neurons from the macula of the utricle join the primary afferent neurons from the cristae of the horizontal and superior semicircular canals to form the superior vestibular nerve. The primary afferent neuron from

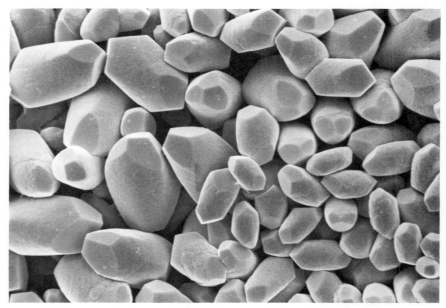

Figure 7–5. Utricular otoconia. (× 3000.) (Courtesy of Charles G. Wright.)

the crista of the posterior semicircular canal (singular nerve) joins the primary afferent neurons from the macula of the saccule to form the inferior division of the vestibular nerve. The cell bodies for all primary afferent neurons are located in Scarpa's ganglion, which is medial to the vestibular labyrinth within the internal auditory canal.

The central processes of the primary vestibular neurons enter the brainstem and synapse in the various vestibular nuclei (superior, lateral, medial, and descending). From these nuclei, neural projections either go through the reticular formation or, in some cases, go directly to several integrated systems. Connections with the cortical centers result in the conscious appreciation of vertigo, whereas connections with the oculomotor system result in a specific pattern of eye movements, with a slow and fast component (nystagmus). Nystagmus is the objective sign of the subjective symptom of vertigo. This rhythmic motion can be measured and recorded by electronystagmography and used as a diagnostic clinical tool.

The sweating and pallor that accompany vertigo result from vestibular projections to the sympathetic nervous system, whereas nausea and vomiting result from involvement of the nucleus ambiguous and phrenic nucleus. Excessive salivation may occur with stimulation of the salivatory nuclei, and connections with the cerebellum and anterior horn cells result in ataxia and postural change. These latter findings are clinically important and can be studied by postural tests (e.g., Romberg) and tests of coordination (e.g., dysdiadochokinesia, finger to nose) (Fig. 7–6).

Diagnosis

The history obtained from a patient with dysequilibrium should be a composite of the different possible diagnoses and, if thorough, will lead to the correct diagnosis in over 80 per cent of the patients. The initial step in the history is to clarify the terminology in an effort to ascertain the exact nature

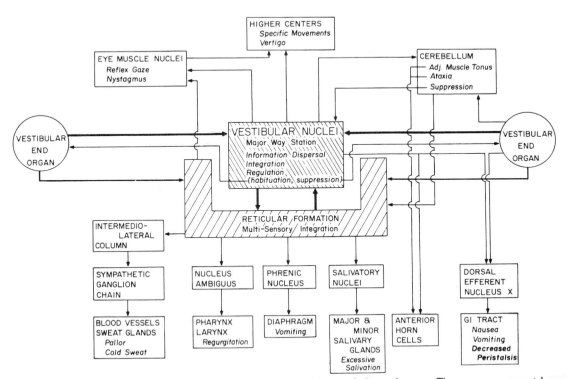

Figure 7–6. Schematic representation of the central projections for vestibular end organ. The arrows represent known tracts. This indicates the high degree to which the vestibular system is integrated into the neuraxis. Under normal circumstances, the vestibular system is principally a proprioceptive one (upper half of schema), but under abnormal circumstances, it initiates considerable motor activity (lower half of schema). (From McCabe BF: Vestibular physiology: its clinical application in understanding the dizzy patient. *In* Paparella MM, Shumrick DA (eds): Otolaryngology. Philadelphia, WB Saunders Company, 1973.)

of the complaint (e.g., vertigo, lightheaded-ness, ataxia, syncope). Once this has been accomplished, the physician should determine the onset, duration, and frequency of symptoms, any precipitating factors (e.g., position change, meals), and associated symptoms. The latter include the aural symptoms of tinnitus, fullness, otorrhea, pain, and hearing loss; the vegetative symptoms of nausea, vomiting, and diaphoresis; and symptoms of disease states known to cause vertigo. One should seek evidence of inflammatory disease, ocular disorders, hypothyroidism, diabetes mellitus, arteriosclerotic vascular disease, allergy, trauma, multiple sclerosis, and toxins (e.g., medications, pollutants).

A complete neurotologic and head and neck examinations are mandatory, with special emphasis on proprioception, balance (Romberg) and gait, cranial nerve function, auscultation for bruits, tuning fork tests, and otoscopy (with the pneumatic otoscope), as well as a general physical examination to identify systemic disease.

Audiologic assessment will identify and quantify associated hearing loss and help to establish the site of lesion. Electronystagmography provides an objective recording of nystagmus and can record eye movement in the dark or with the eyes closed. It also serves as a permanent record of spontaneous nystagmus or that induced by position change, optokinetics, and caloric stimulation. Electronystagmography is a technique in which electrodes record the electric potential difference between the cornea and retina to detect eye movement. This information is then transferred to a polygraph. A characteristic saw-tooth appearance is typical of the saccadic eye movements of nystagmus. By convention, eye deflections to the right are plotted as upward movements and those to the left are plotted as downward movements. The direction of the nystagmus is described as the direction of the fast phase, although physiologically the slow phase is due to the abnormal vestibular input and the fast phase is a correction in eye movement induced by the brainstem.

Caloric tests with either warm and cool air or water are used to induce nystagmus from each ear, following which the nystagmus generated by stimulating the two ears is compared. The results of this comparison may help to identify any abnormalities in the vestibular portion of cranial nerve VIII. In addition, central nervous system causes

of nystagmus can often be differentiated from peripheral (vestibular) causes of nystagmus. Central causes of nystagmus tend to be associated with calibration overshoot, poor eye tracking, optokinetic abnormalities, and lack of suppression of the nystagmus on visual fixation. Nystagmus with position change may occur with either a peripheral or central lesion, although that caused by a peripheral lesion usually has a delay in onset of about 15 to 20 seconds, is not direction changing, is associated with vestibular symptoms, and fatigues with repeated testing, whereas the opposite is true of nystagmus of central origin. Rotational tests with computer analysis may be used as an adjunct and allow testing with a quantifiable stimulus. Such tests as well as vestibulospinal studies and posturography are available only in certain centers but may be of value in difficult cases.

A fluorescent treponemal antibody-absorption test (FTA-abs) will aid in the diagnosis of neurosensory syphilis and should be obtained for all adult patients complaining of vertigo in which the diagnosis is not otherwise obvious. Radiographic evaluation, especially using computed tomography with contrast studies will help identify space-occupying lesions and should be ordered when there is a high index of suspicion. Similarly, cerebrospinal fluid evaluation and hematologic, coagulation, metabolic, chemical, and biochemical studies on the serum should be ordered when suggested by the patient's history and physical examination. An exploratory tympanotomy is usually diagnostic of oval window annular and round window membrane perilymph leaks and may be therapeutic with repair of the leak.

VESTIBULAR DISORDERS

Peripheral causes of rotatory vertigo are much more common than central causes. In most cases, vertigo is the result of a unilateral disorder that results in paresis or paralysis (less commonly, excitation) of the right or left vestibular system with subsequent disproportionate and unequal neural input into the central system. However, disorders of the central system may also result in vertigo.

INFLAMMATORY DISEASES

Microbes

Microbial involvement of the vestibular system may be peripheral or central, and depending on the locus of disease and on whether bacteria, fungi, viruses, or spirochetes are the infecting microorganisms, the clinical manifestations will vary greatly.

Bacterial Infections. Although bacterial labyrinthitis has become quite rare with the advent of antimicrobials, inner ear sequelae as a result of bacterial infections still occur. Bacterial labyrinthitis most frequently occurs as a complication of bacterial meningitis (meningogenic labyrinthitis), with extension of infection to the inner ear through the internal auditory canal or cochlear aqueduct. The clinical course can be catastrophic, with sudden incapacitating vertigo, tinnitus, and profound permanent sensorineural deafness. These symptoms are usually accompanied by nausea and vomiting, diaphoresis, and, frequently, dehydration. Although less common than meningogenic labyrinthitis, bacterial labyrinthitis may be tympanogenic (due to otitis media) or hematogenic (secondary to septicemia). In meningogenic and tympanogenic labyrinthitis, the most frequent offending organism is *Streptococcus pneumoniae*. The sudden onset of severe vertigo and vomiting in association with an otitis media, meningitis, or septicemia suggests that there is suppuration within the inner ear. These symptoms are associated with a brisk nystagmus, which may be irritative (toward the involved ear) early in the course of the disease process but rapidly becomes paralytic (away from the involved ear).

Far less catastrophic than bacterial labyrinthitis, but more frequent in occurrence, is the serous (sterile) labyrinthitis, which occurs secondary to the passage of toxic products of otitis media into the inner ear through the semipermeable round window membrane. This complication may also occur secondary to bony erosion from cholesteatoma or granulation tissue in chronic otitis media. High-frequency sensorineural hearing loss is the usual sequela of this problem, but vestibular disturbance may also occur. The vertigo from serous labyrinthitis is usually much less dramatic than that from bacterial suppurative labyrinthitis, and although some sensorineural hearing loss may occur, the hearing is more likely to recover. The direction of the nystagmus in serous labyrinthitis is usually toward the affected ear (irritative).

Treatment of bacterial labyrinthitis includes hospitalization, appropriate antimicrobial therapy based on culture, fluid replacement, and vestibular suppressants (e.g., Valium, antihistamines). When bacterial labyrinthitis is secondary to acute purulent otitis media, a myringotomy should be performed in addition to the previously described medical treatment. When bacterial labyrinthitis is due to chronic otitis media, a mastoidectomy should be performed as soon as the patient is stable. If these patients do not die from intracranial complications, the catastrophic vertigo will subside in about 5 to 7 days, although the patient will have constant dysequilibium for 6 to 8 weeks and dysequilibium with position change for 6 months and possibly indefinitely. Usually, the older the patient, the longer the symptoms persist. Vestibular response and hearing are usually totally lost in the affected end-organ. Serous labyrinthitis follows a more benign course, and once the middle ear problem is corrected, balance should return and hearing will often return to the premorbid level. Bacterial meningitis may also cause a basal arachnoiditis, with adhesions especially in the cerebellopontine angle. These adhesions may cause a sensorineural hearing loss and may also involve the vestibular nerves with resultant vertigo. In these conditions, *Hemophilus influenzae* is the most common infectious agent.

Viral Agents. The same mechanism by which viral agents cause sensorineural hearing loss exists in virus-induced vertigo. There is no specific treatment for these conditions, the hearing loss may be permanent (about 40 per cent of cases), and the vertigo gradually improves over a several-week period. Neuronitis or ganglionitis is a condition in which the nerve or ganglion itself is actually infected. The most commonly identified virus in these conditions is herpes zoster, and the symptom complex that occurs when it involves the geniculate ganglion is known as the Ramsay Hunt syndrome. This syndrome includes aural pain, facial nerve paralysis, sensorineural hearing loss, vertigo, and a zoster eruption on the pinna, external auditory canal, or palate. Recent histopathologic findings of intraneural and perineural round cell infiltration of the seventh and eighth cranial nerves at the brainstem have raised questions regarding the exact pathophysiology of this condition. Although there is no universally accepted mode of treating herpes zoster oticus, it is important to protect the exposed cornea if the face is paralyzed, and some authors believe that a course of steroids may improve the pain and facial nerve prognosis.

Vestibular nerve mononeuronitis is probably also caused by a viral infection. The clinical pattern is that of an upper respiratory tract infection followed by severe vertigo, nystagmus, nausea, vomiting, diaphoresis, and a unilateral nonreactive vestibular system. Hearing remains normal. The clinical picture gradually improves over some weeks, although hyporeactivity or nonreactivity of that vestibular system to caloric stimulation remains. There is documentation in the literature suggesting the possibility of recurrent episodes on the same side. The treatment of vestibular neuritis is symptomatic (vestibular depressants, bed rest, fluids), with no specific treatment available.

Endolymphatic labyrinthitis is another mechanism by which viruses may cause vertigo. The virus (mumps, rubella, rubeola, or influenza) actually invades the endolymphatic system and damages the membranous end-organ. Presenting symptoms are similar to those of vestibular neuronitis, although sensorineural hearing loss is an additional manifestation of this condition.

A third mechanism by which viruses cause vertigo is perilymphatic labyrinthitis. The usual viral offender in this condition is herpes zoster. Perilymphatic labyrinthitis is much less common than endolymphatic labyrinthitis, the clinical course is indistinguishable and the treatment is the same (supportive). Lastly, most viral agents are capable of causing occlusion of the small vessels of the labyrinth, resulting in sudden sensorineural hearing loss and vertigo. The virus attacks the endothelial cells of the blood vessel wall, causing edema and disruption. It also causes red blood cell disruption, vasoconstriction, platelet agglutination, and hypercoagulation, with subsequent decrease in blood flow and end-organ ischemia. The diagnosis of these viral conditions is primarily on the basis of their historical association with other viral syndromes. The symptoms usually improve once the viral illness resolves, although the hearing loss may be permanent. Viral cultures on stool and cerebrospinal fluid as well as convalescent serum titers will be confirmatory. Unfortunately, no specific therapy is available.

Fungal Agents. Fungi cause vertigo much in the same way as do bacteria. Fungal labyrinthitis, however, occurs only in immunologically depressed and debilitated patients. The microorganisms most commonly involved are *Cryptococcus* sp., *Blastomyces* sp., *Mucor* sp., and *Candida* sp. These organisms gain access to the inner ear by meningogenic, tympanogenic, and hematogenic routes (Fig. 7–7). This type of infection has become more common with the widespread use of chemotherapy and immunobiologic suppressants. In spite of aggressive chemotherapeutic treatment (e.g., amphotericin B), the fungal infection may be the terminal event in these patients.

Spirochetes. Syphilitic labyrinthitis is most common in both the tertiary acquired and congenital forms of the disease, although luetic labyrinthitis may occur as a complication of syphilitic meningoencephalitis, a catastrophic condition that occasionally accompanies the secondary stage of syphilis. Every patient with a rapidly progressive hearing loss (often with fluctuation)

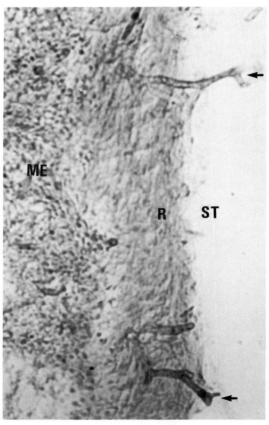

Figure 7–7. *Mucor* sp. (arrows) passing from middle ear (ME) to scala tympani (ST) through round window membrane (R). (× 150.)

with or without vestibular symptoms must be evaluated for luetic infection. The osteitis of the petrous bone that accompanies this disease can cause a perilymphatic fistula, which is responsible for the positive Hennebert's sign (the occurrence of vertigo and nystagmus with pressure application to a sealed external auditory canal and an intact drumhead). Similar to Hennebert's sign, but seen less commonly is the Tullio phenomenon, that is, vertigo with loud noise exposure. The vertigo associated with syphilis may be episodic and may not be very severe. It is important to diagnose this condition, since it may be associated wtih sudden hearing loss. It is thought that this sudden hearing loss can be prevented or reversed by the use of steroids and long-term penicillin. Spirochetes have been identified in the inner ear fluids of these patients and are extremely difficult to eradicate. If indeed the hearing loss is reversed by steroid therapy, this therapy may need to be continued indefinitely.

Allergy

Allergic diatheses (both to inhalants and foods) may be responsible for a number of vertiginous conditions, including Meniere's syndrome. Many patients can identify the allergen that provides the symptoms, but in other patients, an extensive allergic investigation is required. Treatment is hyposensitization or avoidance of the offending allergen, and it is usually successful in controlling the vertigo and associated hearing loss.

VASCULAR AND HEMATOLOGIC DISORDERS

Any condition that results in decreased blood flow to the vestibular end-organ may also result in vertigo. The condition may be caused by a mechanical disorder, systemic disorder (e.g., anemia, leukemia), or altered physiology and may be located as distant from the ear as the heart (e.g., aortic insufficiency) or as close as the internal auditory canal (e.g., anterior vestibular artery thrombosis).

Vascular Disorders

Decreased vascular perfusion as seen with postural change is a frequent cause of dizziness and lightheadedness, inconveniencing the elderly patient who suffers from arteriosclerotic vascular disease and other circulatory problems. Other vascular disorders resulting in vertigo are less common but often associated with more morbidity.

Vertebrobasilar artery insufficiency (VBI) occurs most commonly when the neck is extended or during strenuous exercise with the upper extremities. These activities diminish the blood flow in the vertebrobasilar system, causing a neurologic symptom complex that may range from positional lightheadedness to sudden vertigo with nausea, vomiting, visual field defects, diplopia, headaches, and, sometimes, drop attacks. Conditions resulting in VBI include arteriosclerotic vascular disease (by far the most common), arteritis obliterans, embolism, and polycythemia vera. Vertigo may be a feature of transient ischemic attacks, and patients with these attacks may also have episodes of sudden falling. In cases in which major vessels are stenosed, endarterectomies may improve the cerebral blood flow. Generally, however, the symptoms persist or get worse with time, and patients with this condition should be instructed to try and avoid situations known to precipitate the transient dysequilibrium, especially sudden position change. Vasodilators (e.g., papaverine hydrochloride, nylidrin hydrochloride) may be of some therapeutic value.

The Wallenberg syndrome is a severe neurologic disorder with a very abrupt onset. It is caused by vascular occlusions of the posterior inferior cerebellar artery. This condition results in ischemia of the brainstem and results in devastating neurologic sequelae, including severe vertigo, nausea and vomiting, diplopia, dysphagia, dysphonia, facial weakness, ipsilateral Horner's syndrome, the loss of the sensation of the ipsilateral side of the face and contralateral side of the body, and occasionally, death. There may be a very specific type of nystagmus associated with these symptoms, which is directed toward the side of the lesion when the eyes are closed and away from the side of the lesion when the eyes are open. The diagnosis is made on the basis of the neurologic findings detailed previously. As may be expected with a brainstem infarct, the prognosis is poor.

Migraine is another vascular phenomenon. Although best known as a type of headache, it is also occasionally accompanied by the prodromic signs of severe vertigo, ataxia, tinnitus, and dysarthria. The vasoconstriction in this stage of migraine probably takes place in the basilar artery. In some patients, the hemicranial headache is not as troublesome as the vertigo. Medical treatment of migraine with beta-blockers or other drugs can help decrease the number of vertiginous attacks.

Cerebellar infarcts are being recognized more commonly as a cause of severe vertigo because of the use of computerized axial tomography in diagnosis. Many patients that previously may have been diagnosed as having vestibular neuronitis are now recognized as having small cerebellar infarcts. Large infarcts of the cerebellum present with the typical features of a cerebellar lesion, but small infarcts require a computerized axial tomogram for diagnosis. This test is often performed to exclude cerebellopontine angle lesions, with the cerebellar infarct being a fortuitous finding. Treatment is supportive, and true vertigo should subside within several weeks. Gait disturbance and dysequilibrium often remain as permanent sequelae of cerebellar infarcts.

In general, the diagnosis of vascular insufficiency as the cause of balance disturbance is made on the basis of the patient history. Vertigo secondary to vascular insufficiency is unusual in patients without other evidence of hypertensive heart disease or arteriosclerotic vascular disease, and the episodes usually occur with postural change. Treatment, although of limited value, consists of vasodilators (papaverine hydrochloride, nylidrin hydrochloride) and avoidance of the offending position change. Treatment for the more catastrophic vascular occlusions is directed toward life support and anticoagulation.

Hematologic Disorders

Leukemia, pernicious anemia, and hypercoagulable states have all been associated with vertigo. Leukemia not only decreases the oxygen-carrying capacity of the blood, resulting in end-organ hypoxia, but also frequently involves the petrous apex of the temporal bone with leukemic infiltrate. Hemorrhage into the labyrinth may occur, causing the abrupt onset of roaring tinnitus, incapacitating vertigo, nystagmus, and sudden sensorineural hearing loss. Treatment is supportive, with vestibular suppressants and hydration.

The labyrinthine symptomatology of a hy-percoagulable state can also occur quite suddenly when thrombosis of critical vessels occurs. The symptoms are similar to those of vestibular neuronitis, and therapy is supportive. The dysequilibrium that occurs with various anemias, however, is more subtle and is due to the decreased oxygen-carrying capacity of the blood. This results in end-organ ischemia and dysequilibrium, which occurs primarily with position change. In pernicious anemia, the loss of proprioception makes the dysequilibrium additionally troublesome. The diagnosis of these hematologic conditions is confirmed with hematologic studies (e.g., hemoglobin [Hgb], hematocrit [Hct], peripheral smear).

NEOPLASMS

Primary and metastatic neoplasms located in the cerebellopontine angle, temporal lobe, and cerebellum may all result in dysequilibrium. By far the most common lesion of the cerebellopontine angle associated with dysequilibrium is the acoustic neuroma, although meningiomas, facial nerve schwannomas, vascular abnormalities, metastatic neoplasms, and congenital cholesteatomas may occur. These lesions usually present with an asymmetric high-frequency sensorineural hearing loss and tinnitus. Vertigo or, more commonly, gait disturbance is a later symptom. Acoustic neuromas are unilateral, except in the case of the autosomal dominant syndrome of von Recklinghausen. Much less frequent than cerebellopontine angle lesions are neoplasms of the cerebellum and temporal lobe. The diagnosis of almost all intracranial neoplasms is now made by computed tomography, angiography, nuclear magnetic resonance studies, or contrast radiography. These studies should be obtained if a high index of suspicion is present. Electronystagmography, brainstem response audiometry, and routine audiometry can also provide diagnostic information in this regard. Treatment is usually surgical, although radiation therapy may play a role in selective cases.

TRAUMA

A variety of traumatic conditions may result in vertigo. These include head, neck, and surgical trauma and the trauma associated with sudden implosive and explosive pressure changes (e.g., sneezing, straining, nose blowing). Depending on the severity of the injury, the lesion may be permanent or temporary, minimal or catastrophic.

Temporal Bone Fractures

Temporal bone fractures (a type of basilar skull fracture) are the result of severe head trauma and may be transverse or longitudinal, or a combination of the two (see Chapter 2). Transverse temporal bone fractures transect the nerves of the internal auditory canal or fracture through the labyrinth itself. The result is total sensorineural hearing loss, severe vertigo, and, often, facial nerve paralysis. The diagnosis is suspected following a history of severe head trauma, with subsequent vertigo, nausea, and vomiting. Physical examination will reveal ipsilateral facial nerve paralysis in 50 per cent of patients, hemotympanum, and paralytic nystagmus (away from the involved side). Vertigo is initially treated with vestibular suppressants (e.g., Valium) and hydration. With time, central compensation will physiologically terminate both vertigo and nystagmus. This is a brainstem phenomenon and, depending on age, may require up to 2 weeks. Dysequilibrium, especially with position change, may last 6 to 8 months. Longitudinal temporal bone fractures do not ordinarily involve the vestibular nerve or the labyrinth and, therefore, are not characteristically associated with vertigo. Basilar skull fractures are difficult to identify on plain skull x-rays but are well displayed by hypocycloidal polytomography and computed tomography.

Head Trauma Without Fracture

Head trauma without temporal bone fracture may also cause vertigo, and in some cases, positional vertigo may persist indefinitely. Several theories have been proposed to help explain this phenomenon. It has been demonstrated that head trauma can result in bleeding into the labyrinthine fluids, with subsequent sterile labyrinthitis and vertigo. In this condition, nystagmus toward the involved ear may be the only clinical finding. The course is usually self-limiting, with the nystagmus and vertigo disappearing within 7 to 10 days and the subsequent dysequilibrium, which occurs especially with rapid position change, lasting up to 6 to 8 months. Early in the course, vestibular suppressants may provide symptomatic relief.

An additional explanation for vertigo following head trauma is that of cupulolithiasis. Theoretically, the head trauma dislodges an otoconium from the macula utriculi. Having a relatively high specific gravity, this particle settles in the most dependent portion of the vestibule (ampulla of the posterior semicircular canal). With position change, it rolls onto the cupula of the posterior semicircular canal ampulla, making this a gravity-dependent organ, with resultant vertigo and rotatory nystagmus with position change (benign paroxysmal positional nystagmus). This type of nystagmus is delayed 15 to 20 seconds after position change, is directed toward the involved ear when it is in the down position, fatigues with repeated attempts to elicit it, and is often associated with vertigo, diaphoresis, and nausea. The diagnosis of cupulolithiasis is suspected following a history of head trauma and confirmed with this latter physical finding. Treatment is directed toward hastening central compensation by having the patient repeatedly assume the position that results in paroxysmal positional nystagmus. If this fails and the symptoms persist for more than 1 year, surgical section of the singular nerve (afferent supply from the ampulla of the posterior semicircular canal) may be employed; this procedure is successful in over 80 per cent of cases (Fig. 7–8).

Perilymph Leak

Perilymph leakage from the round window membrane or oval window anulus may occur spontaneously but more commonly follows relative pressure changes between the atmosphere, middle ear, and cerebrospinal fluid. Such pressure changes occur with flying, diving, sneezing, straining, and coughing. The trauma from such pressure changes on the round window membrane or oval window anulus results in perilymph leakage. Classically, the diagnosis is based on the history of sudden pressure change followed by fluctuant hearing loss, vertigo, and often tinnitus. However, the presentation may be quite atypical, with either vertigo or hearing loss occurring as the only symptom and with no antecedent history of sudden pressure change. Results of physical examination may be negative or reveal a positive fistula test. If the tissue does not reseal, stopping the leak, on bed rest with elevation of the head of the bed, surgical

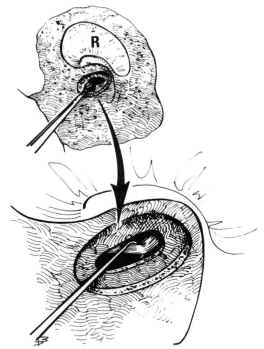

Figure 7–8. Singular nerve section. Area below round window membrane (R) is drilled away to expose singular nerve. The nerve is then avulsed with a small hook.

closure should be considered. A high index of suspicion must be maintained to correctly diagnose this disorder.

Iatrogenic Trauma

Any time the inner ear is entered surgically, either purposefully or inadvertently, damage to the membranous labyrinth may occur with sensorineural hearing loss and vertigo. Upon recognition, such an opening should be sealed with autogenous connective tissue.

Cervical Injury

Cervical spine trauma may be associated with vertigo. Cervical vertigo is a poorly understood entity that occasionally follows flexion-extension or extension-flexion injuries to the neck. Although usually temporary, vertigo with neck torsion may be persistent. Treatment of the vertigo is identical to the orthopedic treatment for the neck injury (soft cervical collar, physiotherapy, muscle relaxants). Vestibular depressants may be of temporary value.

TOXIC AGENTS

Many agents, some pharmacologic and others pollutants, cause dysequilibrium. Of the medicinal items, birth control pills, aminoglycoside antimicrobials, and antihypertensives are most common. The dysequilibrium associated with birth control pills occurs without hearing loss and is reversible with cessation of the medication. Aminoglycoside antimicrobials, on the other hand, usually cause irreversible hearing loss and vestibular damage (Figs. 7–9 to 7–11). This side effect is dose related, dependent on renal function, and enhanced by the presence of other ototoxic drugs. Vestibular damage precedes the hearing loss in the case of streptomycin and gentamicin, whereas the opposite is true with most of the other aminoglycosides. A good deal of research effort is being devoted to developing effective aminoglycoside antimicrobials that have less ototoxicity.

Although the pathophysiology of benign paroxysmal positional nystagmus is poorly understood, this disorder can occasionally occur spontaneously or during ototoxic drug treatment. Pollutants such as alcohol, tobacco, carbon monoxide, and heavy metals (e.g., lead and mercury) may also cause vertigo as a result of their effect on the vestibular nerve or the membranous vestibular labyrinth.

METABOLIC ABNORMALITIES

Certain metabolic abnormalities cause not only sensorineural hearing loss but also vertigo.

Hypothyroidism

It has been estimated that up to 15 per cent of patients with Meniere's disease are hypothyroid and that the Meniere symptoms in one third of these patients will improve with thyroid hormone replacement therapy. The pathophysiology involved is poorly understood, and the endolymphatic hydrops of Meniere's disease has never been observed in experimental hypothyroid animals. Most patients with audiovestibular complaints related to hypothyroidism have other more obvious symptoms, such as weight gain, dry skin, alopecia, and constipation, making the history and physical examination crucial for even suspecting the diagnosis. Laboratory studies will confirm

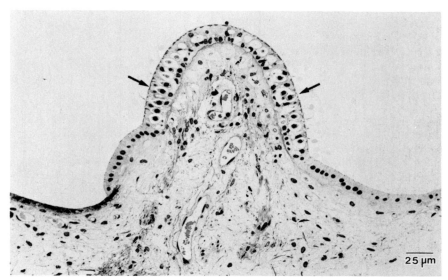

Figure 7–9. Crista ampullaris from an animal sacrificed 14 days after administration of Cortisporin to the middle ear showing loss of hair cells at the crest of the crista and degenerating hair cells on the slopes (arrows). (Courtesy of Charles G. Wright and William L. Meyerhoff.)

the suspicion and guide the treatment with replacement thyroid hormone.

Diabetes Mellitus

Diabetes mellitus is another metabolic aberration associated with dysequilibrium. Aside from postprandial hypoglycemia, several other mechanisms are presumed for this association. Small vessel alterations in the inner ear have been identified in diabetic patients. These alterations include the deposition of periodic acid–Schiff positive material on the vessel walls and aneurysmal dilatations of the capillaries, resulting in local ischemia.

The primary neuropathy known to occur with diabetes mellitus could presumably affect the vestibular nerves, as could the secondary neuropathy due to abnormalities of the vasonervorum. Lastly, the alterations in inner ear glucose concentration that occur in diabetes mellitus affect inner ear function, since inner ear homeostasis is dependent on

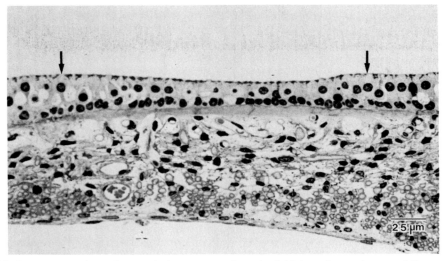

Figure 7–10. Cross section of utricular macula from an animal sacrificed 14 days after application of Cortisporin to middle ear cavity. Hair cells are present in the peripheral positions of the macula (arrows) but are missing in the thinner central area of the neuroepithelium. (Courtesy of Charles G. Wright and William L. Meyerhoff.)

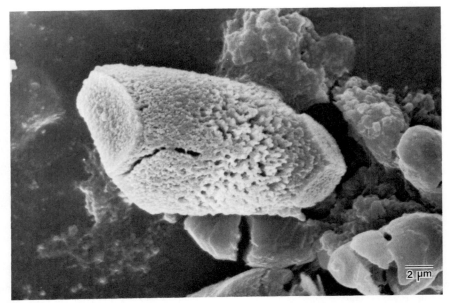

Figure 7–11. Scanning electron micrograph showing degenerating saccular otoconia from an animal sacrificed 14 days after Cortisporin administration. (Courtesy of Charles G. Wright and William L. Meyerhoff.)

normal glucose metabolism. It is not unusual for patients with severe insulin-dependent diabetes to have "multiple sensory deficit," including decreased proprioception and visual loss, compounding the problem.

The diagnosis of diabetes mellitus may be suspected in those patients with a positive family history and polydipsia and polyuria. The diagnosis is confirmed by measuring blood sugar concentrations in the fasting state. The possible treatments for this disorder include dietary discretion, oral hypoglycemics, and insulin. Careful control of glucose metabolism is very effective in controlling the symptom of dysequilibrium, unless the cause is altered proprioception from severe peripheral neuropathy.

Adrenocortical Insufficiency

Adrenocortical insufficiency has been identified as a cause of postural hypotension, resulting in lightheadedness and Meniere's syndrome. The pathophysiology is poorly understood but theories include the following disorders, all of which occur with adrenocortical insufficiency: end-organ hypoxia secondary to vasospasm, abnormal glucose metabolism, lowered serum sodium levels, or alterations of time constants of the neural transmission at the neural junction. The diagnosis requires a high index of suspicion and is confirmed by a measure of the ACTH-stimulated serum cortisol level. Treatment is either with prednisone or physiologic adrenocortical extract and is usually effective in eliminating the vestibular symptoms.

MISCELLANEOUS DISORDERS

Multiple Sclerosis

Multiple sclerosis, or sclerosis multiplex, is known for its fluctuating and often complex symptom pattern. Some symptoms, however, are more frequent than others, and visual problems (e.g., neuronitis retrobulbaris and diplopia) are often the first symptoms of the disease. Vertigo is probably the first symptom in 5 per cent of patients with multiple sclerosis, and during the course of the disease, up to 30 per cent of patients experience vertiginous episodes. Owing to the intranuclear ophthalmoplegia, the nystagmus associated with multiple sclerosis is of a characteristic pattern (dissociated nystagmus on lateral gaze, pendular fixation nystagmus, and an abnormal optokinetic nystagmus) and is often diagnostic on electronystagmography. Brainstem response audiometry often demonstrates abnormalities in patients with multiple sclerosis. The localization of the demyelinization is either in the brainstem or at the entry of the nerve root to the brainstem. Any young patient with bizarre and otherwise unexplained neurologic complaints should be suspected of having multiple sclerosis.

Meniere's Syndrome

This syndrome is a collection of symptoms arising from the peripheral auditory and vestibular systems and includes episodic incapacitating vertigo, fluctuant hearing, aural fullness of pressure, and tinnitus. The severe vertigo usually lasts several hours, following which the patient may be left with tinnitus, aural fullness, and unsteadiness for days. After the initial attacks, the hearing usually returns to normal, but on subsequent occasions, there is a progressive permanent hearing loss. The four symptoms of vertigo, tinnitus, aural fullness, and hearing loss usually occur together, although vertigo may be the first and only symptom leading the observer to initially suspect the diagnosis of vestibular neuronitis. With time, the symptom complex usually becomes complete, establishing the diagnosis of Meniere's syndrome. Occasionally the auditory symptoms of aural fullness, fluctuant hearing, and tinnitus persist by themselves (cochlear Meniere's syndrome) or the episodic incapacitating vertigo may persist by itself (vestibular Meniere's syndrome). A third variant, the syndrome of Lermoyez, involves a different relationship between the auditory acuity and the vestibular attacks. As opposed to Meniere's syndrome, in this syndrome the hearing is improved during and immediately after a vertiginous attack. The fourth varient, the otolithic crisis of Tumarkin, involves sudden falling episodes, due to extensor collapse, without loss of consciousness. There is no well-accepted physiologic explanation for the syndrome of Lermoyez; however, it has been postulated that the otolithic crisis of Tumarkin is caused by membranous ruptures of the saccule or utricle, which had gradually become displaced by hydrops and which, following rupture, undergoes a sudden shift resulting in loss of extensor tone.

The only clinically objective findings in Meniere's syndrome are the presence of nystagmus during an acute attack of vertigo and occasionally a positive Hennebert's sign (nystagmus and vertigo when air pressure is applied against the intact tympanic membrane through a sealed external auditory canal). This phenomenon is due to the adhesions between the stapes footplate and saccule, which occur with endolymphatic hydrops. There are no absolute diagnostic tests for Meniere's syndrome, and although the diagnosis must be made on the history, low-frequency sensorineural hearing loss may be an early clue. With chronicity, the audiogram assumes more of a flat pattern.

Histologically, Meniere's syndrome is characterized by distention of the membranous labyrinth (endolymphatic hydrops) (Fig. 7–12). The cause of this endolymphatic hydrops is unknown, although allergies, vasomotor reactions, trauma, metabolic disor-

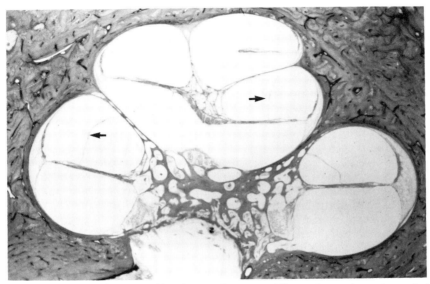

Figure 7–12. Cross section of human cochlea showing distension of Reissner's membrane (arrows). (× 25.)

ders, infectious processes (e.g., viral, syphilitic), hereditary factors, and psychosomatic reactions have all been implicated. The conditions, especially syphilis, thyroid dysfunction, and allergies, should be eliminated as possible etiologic factors before the diagnosis of Meniere's disease (idiopathic endolymphatic hydrops) is made. The diagnosis is then based on the history and supported with audiologic and electronystagmographic testing.

Treatment for Meniere's syndrome with an identifiable cause should be directed toward the cause itself. Treatment for the idiopathic variety (Meniere's disease) includes avoidance of salt, alcohol, nicotine, and caffeine. Diuretics and antivertiginous agents should also be tried. If the medical treatment for Meniere's disease fails, several surgical procedures are available to offer relief from vertigo. For patients with no serviceable hearing, total ablation of inner ear function by a labyrinthectomy or vestibular (eighth cranial) nerve section is very successful. On the other hand, endolymphatic sac decompression, the best surgical procedure reported to control vertigo in a patient with Meniere's disease and serviceable hearing, is one of the most controversial subjects in otology today. In up to 40 per cent of patients, Meniere's disease may involve the contralateral ear.

Cogan's Syndrome

Cogan's syndrome is characterized by the sudden onset of nonsyphilitic interstitial keratitis, episodic vertigo, tinnitus, and profound sensorineural hearing loss. The eye symptoms (pain, photophobia) often precede the ear symptoms, but cases in which the otologic symptoms occur first have been reported. It is believed that Cogan's syndrome is part of a generalized disease process. It has been associated with polyarteritis nodosa and sarcoidosis. Corticosteroids are the treatment of choice.

Bell's Palsy

Idiopathic facial nerve paralysis, Bell's palsy, has recently been identified as having associated sensorineural hearing loss and vertigo in a large number of cases. These last two symptoms can be documented on audiogram and electronystagmography, respectively, and their occurrence has led some

observers to believe that this disorder is merely part of a polyneuropathy. Although the etiology is unknown, viral infection is suspect. The diagnosis of idiopathic facial paralysis can only be made after a thorough examination has excluded other etiologic factors (e.g., tumors, trauma, and middle ear infection) as the cause of the facial nerve paralysis. The site of the facial nerve lesion can be clinically identified. This is extremely important if one contemplates surgical intervention. Lesions central to the facial nucleus spare the upper half of the face from paralysis due to cross innervation at that level. Lesions in the cerebellopontine angle that produce a facial palsy will usually also affect the acoustic nerve and result in sensorineural hearing loss. Lesions central to the geniculate ganglion but peripheral to the brainstem will produce a dry eye owing to interruption of the parasympathetic nerve supply to the lacrimal gland. This can be demonstrated with a Schirmer test, in which a strip of filter paper is placed between the lower lid and sclera of both eyes and tearing with and without ammonia stimulation is measured. Lesions in the horizontal section of the middle ear will eliminate the stapes reflex but preserve tearing, whereas lesions in the mastoid portion, proximal to the chorda tympani, will affect taste, which can be tested with an electrical gustometer, and will also decrease ipsilateral salivary flow while preserving the stapedial reflex. A variety of electrical tests of peripheral nerve function have been devised to follow the progress of the disease. These include the minimal nerve excitability test and electroneuronography. Unfortunately, changes in results of all these tests lag several days behind the actual physiological status of the nerve, and none is absolutely accurate in predicting nerve recovery. Electromyography may be used in conjunction with maximum nerve stimulation or by itself. When used by itself, it may demonstrate fibrillation potentials 10 days to 2 weeks after nerve degeneration. It can also demonstrate recovery potentials at about 21 days if recovery is going to occur. This demonstration of recovery potentials occurs before they become clinically apparent.

The treatment of Bell's palsy is not standarized. Many physicians prescribe corticosteroids, although recent studies have questioned the efficacy of these drugs. Surgical decompression can be performed, but there is a good deal of disagreement about when to perform this surgery and also about how much of the nerve to decompress. Also, there is no well-controlled study showing that decompression improves the ultimate prognosis. One important factor in treating Bell's palsy is to protect the cornea against exposure keratitis. Almost all patients with Bell's palsy recover to a greater or lesser extent. Patients with partial paralysis have a very high degree of recovery. Some physicians elect no therapy at all, since they believe it is of no value and the associated vertigo almost always improves.

Temporal Lobe Epilepsy

The idiopathic phenomenon of temporal lobe epilepsy presents with episodic vertigo in the absence of sensorineural hearing loss. It is usually seen in prepubescent patients, and it has a characteristic electronystagmographic pattern (nystagmus worsens with eyes open). This coupled with an abnormal electroencephalogram is diagnostic. Treatment is with anticonvulsants.

Treatment

MEDICAL MANAGEMENT

When a specific etiology for vertigo can be identified, therapy should be instituted as described in the preceding text. In many cases, however, a specific diagnosis eludes the physician or there is no specific treatment. When this occurs, nonspecific therapy must be employed. The medical treatment in such a case begins with *general measures* concerning the patient's life style. Included among these measures are sufficient rest and judicious exercise, along with the avoidance of stress, alcohol, caffeine, tobacco, spices, salt, and potentially incriminating medications that are not life-supporting (e.g., birth control pills, aspirin, quinine, tranquilizers). There are not many cases of vertigo in which the attack comes on without warning. Nevertheless, the patient may have to make some changes if employment requires working at heights or with moving machinery, or driving or flying.

When the vertiginous attack is acute and incapacitating neuroleptanalgesics (Innovar, 1 ml in 10 ml normal saline given slowly by the intravenous route, and Valium, 10 to 20 mg, given slowly by the intravenous route)

are very effective in controlling the symptoms. The former is a combination drug with fentanyl (narcotic analgesic) and droperidol (tranquilizer). The mode of action in reducing or alleviating vertigo is poorly understood but probably occurs at the level of the central nervous system. Patients must be carefully monitored in a hospital setting for respiratory depression and apnea while receiving these drugs. Valium (diazepam) also has a central calming effect but additionally appears to have a direct suppressant effect on the activity within the vestibular nuclei.

In recurrent attacks of a milder nature, a choice of medications is available. *Diuretics* are frequently prescribed based on the theory that fluid retention plays a role in endolymphatic hydrops, especially when symptoms occur in the premenstrual period. Whether such medications influence inner ear fluid volumes is speculative. The usual dosage of hydrochlorothiazide is 50 mg daily, and the patient should be warned about the need to eat food with high potassium content or to use a potassium supplement. This warning is especially important in patients on digitalis therapy, and serum potassium levels should be measured at quarterly intervals in such patients. *Antihistamines* (e.g., meclizine hydrochloride, Dramamine) are often very effective in reducing subjective vertigo and its associated vegetative symptoms (nausea, vomiting). In addition to their obvious competitive antagonism to histamine, antihistamines have a significant effect on the central nervous system, helping account for their usefulness in the treatment of vertigo, nausea, and vomiting. Although the mechanism of action is not clearly understood, the anticholinergic properties of antihistamines certainly play a role. A frequent and disturbing side effect of antihistamines, however, is somnolence, which occurs in about 50 per cent of patients.

Anticholinergic therapy can be offered to the patient in the form of sublingual scopolamine, especially in anticipation of an attack. The sublingual placement of 0.4 mg seems to be helpful in avoiding vertiginous attacks in certain patients. Transcutaneous scopolamine delivered from an adhesive patch worn behind the ear is a very convenient method of controlling vertigo and motion sickness. Side effects of dry mouth, blurred vision, and palpitations must be discussed with the patient. Scopolamine (0.6

mg) can also be used in combination with D-amphetamine (10 mg) as an oral preparation to decrease both subjective vertigo and nausea and vomiting. The physician using this combination must be alert to the addicting properties of D-amphetamine.

Vasodilators have been used for almost all inner ear symptoms, and vertigo is no exception. The smooth muscle relaxants (nylidrin hydrochloride, papaverine hydrochloride) are most effective in increasing blood flow to the peripheral labyrinth and may be used on an outpatient basis. For hospitalized patients, 5 per cent CO_2 mixed with 95 per cent O_2 administered for 30 minutes four times daily, is very effective. When vascular insufficiency is the underlying cause of balance disturbance, vasodilators may be quite helpful. Lastly, *vestibulotoxic* drugs can be administered to patients suffering from vertigo originating from the peripheral labyrinth. Both streptomycin and gentamicin are aminoglycoside antimicrobials that functionally ablate the vestibular end-organ prior to causing noticeable hearing loss. These ototoxic drugs can be given systemically or by way of catheter infusion into the middle ear. In the latter case, the drug passes across the round window membrane, resulting in a unilateral ablative effect. However, with this form of drug administration, hearing is at significant risk. Patients should be hospitalized for this treatment and carefully monitored with electronystagmography and audiology. They should also be monitored for changes in renal function.

SURGICAL MANAGEMENT

Surgical treatment of vertigo may be specific in such conditions as otosclerosis, endolymphatic hydrops, perilymph fistula, and benign paroxysmal positional vertigo, or it may be nonspecific. Stapedectomy will relieve the occasional vertigo associated with otosclerosis in a certain percentage of patients, and sealing an opening resulting in perilymph leak is highly successful in the presence of that condition. Singular nerve section involves cutting the nerve from the ampulla of the posterior semicircular canal and is successful in relieving vertigo in about 80 per cent of patients suffering benign paroxysmal positional vertigo.

Endolymphatic sac surgery is employed in selected cases of Meniere's disease. The objective of this procedure is to decompress the endolymphatic system by draining it into the mastoid cavity or subarachnoid space. The patient is relieved of vertigo or improved in almost 80 per cent of cases. Additional hearing loss occurs in 3 to 5 per cent of patients as a result of these operations. Cerebrospinal fluid otorrhea and meningitis are potential complications of the endolymphatic sac–subarachnoid procedure. Other decompression procedures for Meniere's disease include trans-stapedial sacculotomy, otic-perotic shunt, and cryosurgery. The former can be accompanied in a repetitive manner by implanting a stainless steel tack through the anterior-inferior aspect of the stapes footplate. This operation enjoys almost certain success in relieving vertigo, but the resulting additional hearing loss is a drawback.

The otic-perotic shunt is a technically difficult surgical procedure that involves placement of an inert shunt tube through the basilar membrane of the cochlea by way of the round window membrane. Theoretically, this tube allows communication between the scala media and scala tympani, with subsequent decompression of the endolymphatic space. In addition to being technically difficult to perform, this procedure is extremely traumatic to the delicate structures of the inner ear and results in a high incidence of sensorineural hearing loss.

Endolymphatic-perilymphatic fistulae can also be created by cryosurgery when the cryoprobe is applied to the round window, promontory, or horizontal semicircular canal. The effect of cryosurgery results from a temperature/time relationship, and requires a specially designed probe tip. The potential of facial nerve paralysis in this procedure is a definite drawback.

Destructive surgical procedures are also used to treat patients who are suffering from vertigo. When hearing is an important consideration, the vestibular division of cranial nerve VIII can be sectioned through the middle cranial fossa (Fig. 7–13). This procedure is technically difficult but results in ablation of vestibular complaints in almost 100 per cent of patients and preserves hearing in 80 per cent of patients. When preservation of hearing is not important, destruction of the peripheral end-organ (semicircular canals and utricle) can be performed by a labyrinthectomy. In this procedure, the membranous labyrinth is actually removed either through the external auditory canal or by

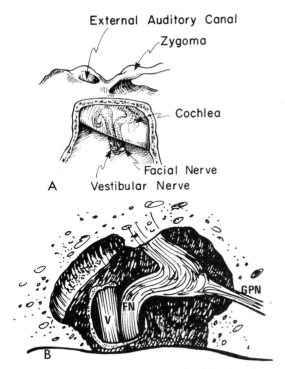

External Auditory Canal

Zygoma

Cochlea

Facial Nerve

A Vestibular Nerve

GPN

FN

V

B

Figure 7–13. *A,* Surgeon's view of middle cranial fossa nerve section. *B,* Closer view of the relationship between the facial nerve (FN), the superior vestibular nerve (V), and the greater petrosal nerve (GPN).

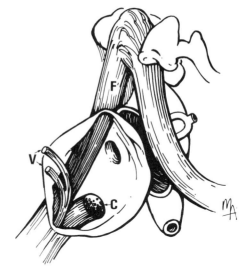

Figure 7–14. Surgeon's view of translabyrinthine eighth nerve section. The facial nerve (F) and the cochlear (C) and vestibular (V) divisions of the eighth nerve can be seen.

the transmastoid route. This procedure is successful in approximately 85 per cent of cases, but because of the additional 15 per cent of cases not helped by this procedure, some clinicians prefer the translabyrinthine eighth nerve section (Fig. 7–14). This latter operation results in complete elimination of peripheral vestibular input. The reason for failure in total labyrinthectomy is not totally understood, but some observers believe that it is due to postsurgical vestibular neuroma formation or incomplete removal of the vestibular end-organ.

Lastly, some clinicians have used ultrasound waves to destroy the membranous vestibular labyrinth. Since these waves pass through various media, they are partially absorbed, depending on the conductivity of the media. As energy is absorbed it is converted to heat and results in biologic changes with eventual tissue destruction.

BIBLIOGRAPHY

Afzelius, L. E., Henriksson, N. G., and Wahlgren, L.: Vertigo and dizziness of functional origin. Laryngoscope 90:649–656, 1980.

Bagger-Sjoback, D., Lundquist, P. G., Galey, F., and Ylikoski, J.: The sensory epithelia of the human labyrinth. Am J Otol 4:203–212, 1983.

Beddoe, G. M.: Vertigo in childhood. Otolaryngol Clin North Am 10:139–144, 1977.

Gacek, R. R.: Vestibular neuroanatomy. Ann Otol Rhinol Laryngol 88:667–675, 1979.

Gacek, R. R.: Neuroanatomical correlates of vestibular function. Ann Otol Rhinol Laryngol 89:2–5, 1980.

Hunter-Duvar, I. M.: An electron microscopic study of the vestibular sensory epithelium. Acta Otolaryngol 95:494–507, 1983.

Jongkees, L. B. W.: Vestibular physiology and tests. Arch Otolaryngol 89:37–44, 1969.

McCabe, B. F.: Vestibular physiology: its clinical application in understanding the dizzy patient. *In* Paparella, M. M., and Shumrick, W. B. (eds.): Otolaryngology, Vol. 1. 2nd ed. Philadelphia, W. B. Saunders Co., 1980.

Meyerhoff, W. L., and Paparella, M. M.: Meniere's disease and its various surgical therapies. Otolaryngol Clin North Am 13:767–773, 1980.

Schuknecht, H. F.: Cupulolithiasis. Arch Otolaryngol 90:113–126, 1969.

Schumacher, G. A.: Demyelinating diseases as a cause for vertigo. Arch Otolaryngology 85:93–94, 1967.

Wolfson, R. J.: Labyrinthine surgery for Meniere's disease. Otolaryngol Clin North Am. 6:131–138, 1973.

Earl R. Harford

8

BASIC AUDIOLOGIC EVALUATION AND REMEDIAL MANAGEMENT OF THE HEARING IMPAIRED

The objective of a basic audiologic evaluation is to obtain quantifiable information on the status of a patient's auditory mechanism and functional hearing efficiency. More specifically, a basic audiologic evaluation should provide an answer to each of the following questions:

1. Is there a loss of auditory sensitivity, and if so, precisely how much?

2. What is the relationship between ears?

3. What is the audiometric configuration for each ear?

4. What type of loss is present in each ear: pure conductive, pure sensorineural, or mixed? If it is sensorineural, can a retrocochlear disorder be ruled out?

5. What is the patient's capacity for processing simple speech?

6. Is the patient a candidate for amplification?

The contemporary basic audiologic evaluation consists of at least pure tone audiometry, speech audiometry, and impedance audiometry. Sometimes it is necessary to employ additional procedures or modifications of these routine tests in order to provide answers to the six basic questions.

The audiologic evaluation should be a part of the initial otologic examination of a patient, which also includes a history and careful physical inspection of the ears, nose, and throat. Also, an audiologic evaluation is a first step in a rehabilitative regimen for a hearing-impaired patient. The audiologic evaluation provides a graphic and numerical description of the status of a patient's peripheral auditory mechanism and hearing function. Audiologic remedial management or rehabilitative process involves professional services and procedures designed to maximize the patient's residual hearing and other sensory modalities for purposes of optimal communication.

The objective of this chapter is to describe the essential components of the basic audiologic evaluation as well as to provide an overview on the topic of amplification for the hearing impaired, which is the logical alternative in the remedial management of patients with irreversible hearing loss.

Available Tests

PURE TONE AUDIOMETRY

Pure tone audiometry involves the use of an electronic instrument for the measurement of auditory sensitivity for discrete acoustic frequencies. This procedure uses as its model the Rinne tuning fork test, which

127

is described in Chapter 1. The pure tone audiometer was introduced in the United States as a commercial product in the early 1920s. At that time, it was a crude device, but it did offer an improvement over tuning fork tests because the intensity of test signals could be determined with greater accuracy. It took nearly 45 years, until the mid 1960s, before the audiometer was truly perfected. Even today, engineers are further refining these instruments, using microprocessors to allow for computerized pure tone audiometry. The principal of pure tone audiometry is the same, whether a manual or computerized instrument is used.

A pure tone audiometer, like that shown in Figure 8–1, offers precise control of the frequency and intensity of a simple sine wave, commonly called a pure tone. Most pure tone audiometers generate at least seven discrete frequencies from 250 to 8000 Hz, or 0.25 kHz to 8 kHz. Typically, they produce these pure tones from an air conduction earphone over a sound pressure range from 7 dB SPL (sound pressure level), which equals 0.0002 dyne per cm², to about 120 dB SPL, depending upon the frequency of the signal. Figure 8–2 shows the schematic or block diagram of the components of the basic pure tone audiometer. Audiometers not designed exclusively for screening purposes provide the capability of driving a bone-conduction oscillator over a frequency range from 250 to 4000 Hz. For technical reasons, the output intensity range of the bone-conduction vibrator is roughly half that of an air-conduction earphone. Audiometers are designed with switches and controls that allow the tester to deliver an air-conduction stimulus to the right or left ear, select air or bone-conduction stimuli, and introduce the signal at any given time for as long as desired. The audiometer shown in Figure 8–1 is a basic portable instrument. Figure 8–3 shows a more complex clinical audiometer. It contains the same basic features as the portable plus many more options for advanced measures of auditory function.

By the mid 1960s, the International Standardization Organization (ISO) established sound pressure levels for each test frequency that represented average normal hearing. These values were adopted throughout the world for uniformity of this measure. Thus, all audiometers now provide essentially the same information on a given person's hearing level. This is analogous to the worldwide use of the metric system. This simply fosters communication and exchange of information with greater ease and less chance for misinterpretation.

When establishing the status of a patient's hearing sensitivity, a relative decibel scale is used, which is referred to as a hearing level scale. Zero dB at each frequency on this scale represents the amount of sound

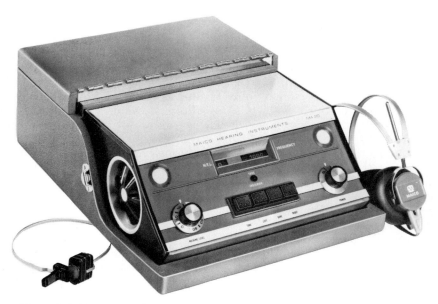

Figure 8–1. Pure tone audiometer. (Courtesy of Maico, Inc., Minneapolis, Minnesota.)

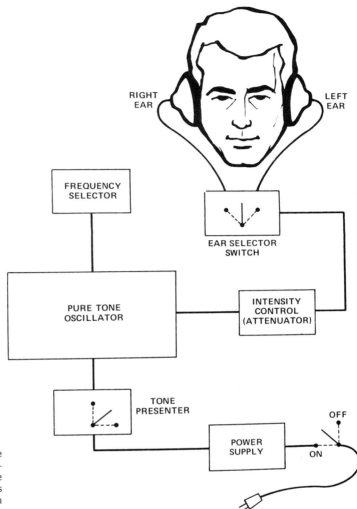

Figure 8–2. Block diagram of a basic pure tone audiometer, showing the essential components necessary to produce simple sine waves and control the output of these signals as they are delivered to an air-conduction earphone or bone-conduction vibrator.

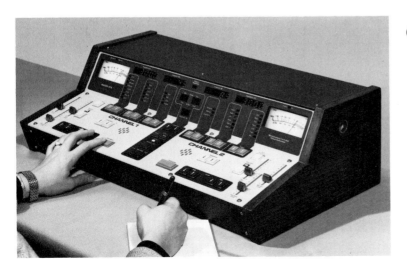

Figure 8–3. Pure tone audiometer. (Grason-Stadler, Model 1701).

pressure necessary for the average normal-hearing young adult to just detect its presence. Thus, each decibel level greater than zero represents a departure from average normal hearing. In pure tone audiometry, the objective is to establish the faintest or lowest hearing level for each test frequency that the patient is just barely able to detect. This is commonly labeled the hearing threshold level (HTL).

Hearing threshold level is plotted on a chart or graph, like that illustrated in Figure 8–4, which is called an audiogram. The numbers across the top of the chart pertain to the frequency of the stimulus in Hertz (Hz) or kilohertz (kHz). The smaller numbers toward the left represent low-pitched sounds, and those to the right are high-pitched sounds. Hearing threshold levels are routinely measured for 250, 500, 2000, 4000, and 8000 Hz. Sometimes, hearing threshold levels are established for 125 Hz as well as 750, 1500, 3000, and/or 6000 Hz.

People with normal hearing will detect all test frequencies at or near 0 dB. The normal range for adults is 0 to 20 dB HL (hearing level). There is mounting evidence that young children cannot afford hearing levels poorer than 10 dB for an extended period of time without some detrimental effects on language, learning development, cognition, and other areas of communication and psychosocial development. Most elements or phonemes of speech fall within the frequency range from 300 Hz to 4000 Hz. Vowels are low-frequency sounds, whereas consonants fall in the mid- and high-frequency ranges. Vowels contain more energy than the weaker consonant sounds. Thus, it is especially important to have good hearing for this range, especially in the higher frequencies. One can have a profound loss of sensitivity above 4 kHz and rarely be aware of abnormal hearing in everyday communication. Figure 8–5 shows a normal audiogram for air-conducted pure tones.

From the early days of pure tone audiometry, a method of "pure tone averaging" has been used to express a patient's degree of loss in hearing sensitivity by a single number for each ear. This technique continues to be used today because it offers a convenient system for describing the degree of hearing loss. To arrive at a pure tone average (PTA), we simply calculate the arithmetic mean of the thresholds for 500, 1000, and 2000 Hz for each ear. Finally, a single value for both ears can be expressed by using a method called the best binaural average (BBA). In this case, the arithmetic average of the better threshold, regardless of ear, is calculated for 500, 100, and 2000 Hz. An

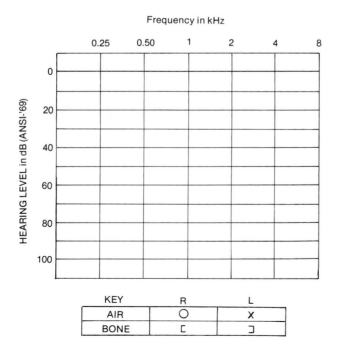

Frequency in kHz

Figure 8–4. Typical graph or audiogram form on which hearing threshold level is recorded.

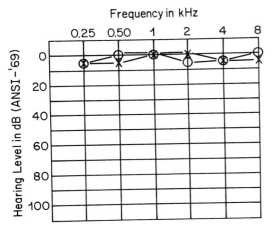

Figure 8–5. An audiogram of a person with normal hearing sensitivity over a range from 250 to 8000 Hz.

example of this averaging is illustrated in Figure 8–6.

Table 8–1 summarizes the classification of the degree of hearing loss according to the author's experience. In other words, there is no standard scale for classifying degree of loss, but the scale in Table 8–1 is realistic. The values and descriptions shown in Table 8–1 might vary slightly by a few decibels if one was to survey a group of audiologists. This table is offered as a guideline for attaching a subjective label (e.g., mild, moderate) to a specific degree of loss, as expressed by the pure tone average for one or both ears.

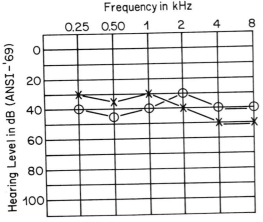

Figure 8–6. Air-conduction audiogram with pure tone averaging shown below:

				Average
Right	45	40	30	38
Left	35	30	40	35
Binaural	35	30	30	32

Recall that pure tone audiometry involves the measurement of hearing sensitivity of two pathways, air conduction and bone conduction. A different type of sound transducer is used for each, as illustrated in Figure 8–7 and 8–8. In testing by air conduction, the stimulus passes through the usual channel from the outer ear to the cochlea. When using bone conduction, the test tone reaches the cochlea by an alternate pathway, mainly bypassing the air-conduction pathway. Probably the middle ear plays some role, but the exact mechanism of bone conduction is still not certain. Comparison of the hearing sensitivity of these two measurements corresponds to the Rinne tuning fork test and helps greatly in determining the gross site of the lesion causing hearing loss. Figures 8–9 to 8–11 illustrate audiometrically the three types of hearing loss: conductive, sensorineural, and mixed.

A pure conductive hearing loss will manifest essentially normal hearing by bone conduction and abnormal hearing by air conduction (see Fig. 8–9). A patient with a pure sensorineural hearing loss (cochlea or eighth cranial nerve disorder) will report essentially the same hearing loss for both air- and bone-conducted tones (see Fig. 8–10). Finally, a patient with a mixed loss will manifest abnormal hearing by both air and bone conduction, but the loss by air conduction will be significantly greater than that by bone conduction (see Fig. 8–11).

Contrary to general assumption, bone conduction is not a true measure of cochlear reserve in patients with a conductive hearing loss. As mentioned earlier, the middle ear structures probably play a role in the transmission of bone-conducted stimuli. A malfunction of this portion of the auditory mechanism can cause a mechanical loss in the transmission of energy from a bone-conduction vibrator to the cochlea. A classic example of this is seen in patients with a stapedial fixation due to otosclerosis. In such cases, we will observe a decrease in hearing sensitivity by bone conduction at 1000 and 2000 Hz, which usually disappears following microsurgery to correct the mechanical malfunction of the ossicular chain. Figure 8–12 shows a typical audiogram of a patient with otosclerosis, which illustrates this mechanical factor in the bone conduction. This pseudoneurosensory hearing loss is referred to as a "mechanical factor" in hearing thresholds of bone conduction. It was first described by Carhart in 1962 and, in the

Table 8–1. CLASSIFICATION OF DEGREE OF HEARING LOSS

Degree	Average Hearing Level for 500, 1000, and 2000 Hz in the Better Ear*		Ability to Detect Speech
	At Least	Less Than	
None	—	25 dB	No difficulty
Slight	25 dB	40 dB	Difficulty with faint speech
Mild	40 dB	55 dB	Frequent difficulty with faint speech
Moderate	55 dB	70 dB	Frequent difficulty with loud speech
Severe	70 dB	90 dB	Can hear only shouted or amplified speech
Profound	90 dB	—	Very limited usable hearing

*1969 ANSI Reference Level

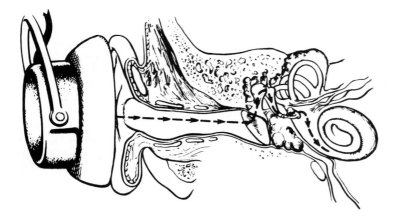

Figure 8–7. An illustration of an air-conduction earphone. Note that the phone is placed directly over the external ear canal, and the sound waves are conducted (by air) to the eardrum and through the middle ear to the inner ear.

Figure 8–8. Sound can be transmitted directly to the inner ear through the bones of the skull by means of a bone-conduction vibrator placed on the mastoid bone behind the outer ear. The broken rule (with arrows) shows the path taken by the sound waves through the bony areas of the head of the inner ear.

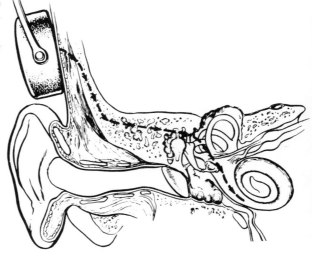

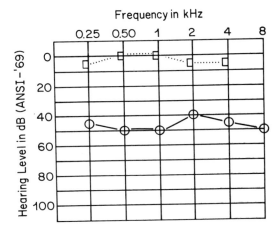

Figure 8–9. An audiogram showing a pure conductive hearing loss.

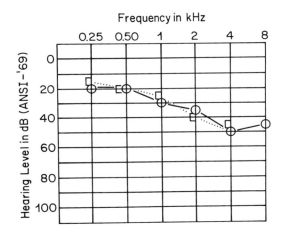

Figure 8–10. An audiogram showing a pure sensorineural hearing loss due to either a cochlear or an eighth nerve disorder.

Figure 8–11. A typical audiogram of a patient with a mixed (conductive and sensorineural) type of hearing loss. There is an air-bone gap, and the bone-conduction thresholds are not within the normal range.

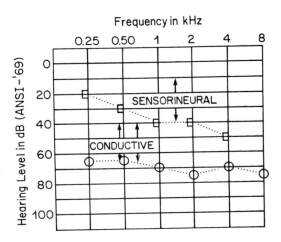

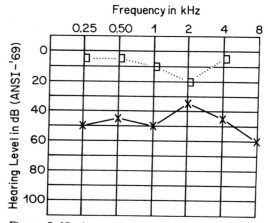

Figure 8–12. A typical preoperative audiogram of a patient with surgically confirmed stapedial otosclerosis.

Pure tone audiometry is the most fundamental procedure provided by audiologists. The audiogram has taken its place as the cornerstone in the study of hearing impairment. This time-honored procedure has multiple applications. It serves as a graphic illustration of the degree of hearing loss, the gross type of loss, the relationship between ears, and the audiometric configuration. The pure tone audiogram offers valuable information about these aspects of the status of a patient's hearing and peripheral hearing mechanism. However, this represents only a portion of the information that should be gathered on a patient. The next step is to measure the patient's capacity to hear and understand controlled-speech stimuli.

SPEECH AUDIOMETRY

Basic speech audiometry provides a measure of two characteristics of hearing for speech stimuli: (1) how loud words must be in order to hear them, and (2) how clearly words are heard when they are loud enough to overcome a loss in hearing sensitivity. Thus, basic speech audiometry consists of two measures: (1) speech threshold, which is analogous to pure tone threshold, and (2) auditory speech discrimination or recognition, which is a measure of the patient's ability to differentiate between the various phonemes of speech at specified levels above the patient's speech threshold or pure tone average. Stated differently, speech audiometry provides a measure of a patient's capacity to receive and process a specified speech message. Pure tone audiometry has major limitations for predicting a patient's functional efficiency in processing speech. Thus, tests that employ standardized speech materials have long been an integral part of the basic audiologic evaluation. In more recent years, speech audiometric tests have been designed to assist in determining a more specific site of lesion (e.g., cochlear versus eighth nerve or brainstem) than is possible with routine pure tone audiometry. Consequently, today, speech audiometry is used as a diagnostic tool as well as an indicator of functional hearing efficiency.

presence of stapedial otosclerosis, is often called the "Carhart Notch." In brief, in conductive hearing loss, bone conduction provides an *estimate* of a patient's cochlear reserve. Bone-conduction measures are more unstable than air-conduction thresholds, especially in conductive hearing loss. At best, bone-conduction audiometry is a relatively weak clinical tool that is subject to considerable variability. It offers a good qualitative measure of the presence of a conductive component, but one should not view bone-conduction thresholds with the same degree of confidence as air-conduction thresholds. Another important point should be made before proceeding. Like most audiometric tests, air- and bone-conduction audiometry are behavioral or inferential measurements, subject to a certain amount of test-retest variability. Over the years, most clinicians and researchers have come to accept a ±5 dB or a 10 dB range of variability from test to test in both air- and bone-conduction thresholds. This point is especially important when comparing the results of two audiograms of the same patient, whether the tests were done on the same day or a year apart.

When hearing threshold levels are recorded on an audiogram and the symbols are connected, the curve that results is called an audiometric configuration. Most hearing losses will fall into a particular classifiable configuration, which can be used, in part, to describe a hearing loss. Examples of the most common audiometric configurations are displayed in Figures 8–13 to 8–20.

Speech Audiometer

Most modern diagnostic or clinical audiometers include the necessary circuitry for both speech and pure tone audiometry. It is unusual to see an instrument that is limited

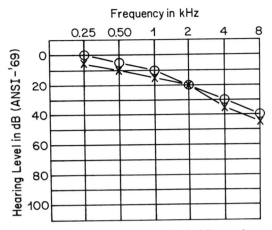

Figure 8–13. An example of a gradually falling audiometric configuration.

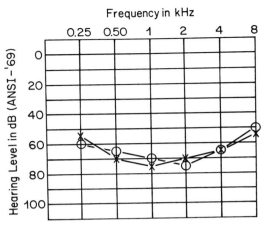

Figure 8–16. An example of a trough-shaped audiometric configuration.

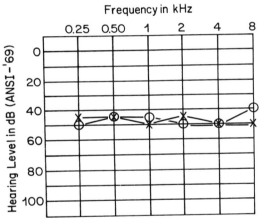

Figure 8–14. An example of a relatively flat audiometric configuration.

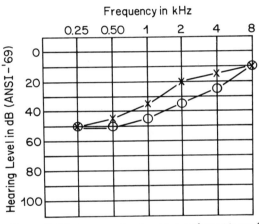

Figure 8–17. An example of a rising audiometric configuration.

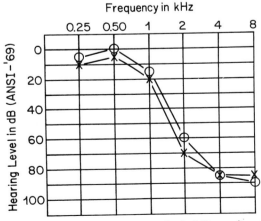

Figure 8–15. An example of a markedly falling audiometric configuration.

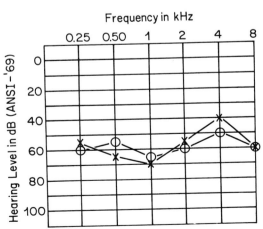

Figure 8–18. An example of a jagged audiometric configuration.

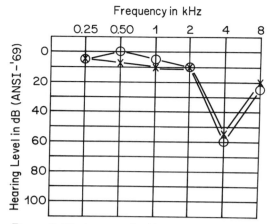

Figure 8–19. An example of a high-frequency notch audiometric configuration.

to speech audiometry. The output of the speech signal, as well as other types of stimuli, can be directed to earphones, a bone vibrator, or to loudspeakers situated in the test room. Most popular diagnostic audiometers contain a two-channel system that allows the audiologist to deliver two types of stimuli or the same stimuli to more than one output transducer (earphone or loudspeaker). This is done to produce a "cocktail party effect" to measure a patient's capacity to handle two or more competing messages. In brief, speech audiometry is a procedure that involves the application of highly controlled speech stimuli to the ear of a patient, just like pure tone audiometry, or from a loudspeaker in an open, acoustically controlled room, as if a person were talking to the patient. In order to do this effectively, it is necessary to use well-calibrated electronic instruments that offer precise control over the stimulus. Equally important is the use of well-standardized test materials, so that the results can be repeated with good reliability.

Speech audiometry can be conducted using earphones or in the sound field (presenting speech from loudspeakers in the test room). Good speech audiometry requires a two-room arrangement so that the patient can be placed in one room alone, with the audiologist and audiometer in an adjoining room. A window between the rooms and an intercommunication system are essential. Figure 8–22 is a schematic of a typical two-room arrangement for performing speech audiometry as well as most pure tone audiometry, especially for older children and adults.

The speech circuit and transducers of a diagnostic audiometer must offer high-fidelity signals and cover a range of about 100 dB. This allows the audiologist to measure the hearing level for speech of patients with various degrees of hearing loss. Like pure tones, speech is also governed by acceptable standards set forth by the American National Standards Institute (ANSI), which also offers precise guidelines for calibration.

to just speech audiometry. Figure 8–21 shows an example of a modern "diagnostic audiometer," which offers the flexibility of pure tone and speech audiometry, as well as more advanced special auditory tests. A similar instrument is shown in Figure 8–3. These instruments contain a number of switches and controls in addition to several types of stimuli for measuring various parameters of the auditory system. These audiometers allow for the input of "live" speech spoken by the audiologist into a microphone. This mode of speech audiometry is called monitored live voice testing. It is possible also to provide the input with speech tests recorded on magnetic tape; this is the most controlled and reliable approach

Speech Reception Threshold

A speech reception threshold (SRT) is the sound intensity level at which a patient is just capable of correctly identifying simple speech stimuli. This level is analogous to a threshold for pure tones and correlates with

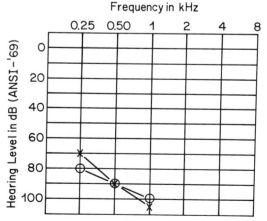

Figure 8–20. An example of a fragmentary audiometric configuration.

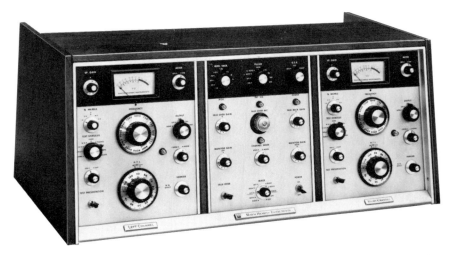

Figure 8–21. Diagnostic audiometer. (Courtesy of Maico, Inc., Minneapolis, Minnesota.)

the pure tone average for 500, 1000, and 2000 Hz. Thus, the SRT serves as an excellent cross check on the validity of pure tone thresholds in the speech frequency range (500 to 2000 Hz). A discrepancy (9 dB or more) between the SRT and pure tone average, with the SRT better than the pure tone average, suggests a functional disorder unless there is a precipitous high-frequency audiometric configuration. Another reason for establishing an SRT is to provide a reference for conducting speech discrimination tests. That is, the SRT is used to calculate the sensation level (SL) for the presentation of speech discrimination materials to determine how well the patient can understand comfortably loud speech (words or sentences). Another reason for using the SRT is to determine the functional gain of a hearing aid for a patient by comparing unaided with aided speech thresholds.

A standardized list of 36 two-syllable words (spondaic words) is used for establishing speech thresholds. This list was developed at the Harvard Psychoacoustic Laboratory in the mid 1940s and has served its purpose well over the years. As stated earlier, the SRT should correlate highly with the pure tone average. Thus, the SRT can be substituted for the pure tone average in Table 8–1, with essentially the same interpretation.

Figure 8–22. Schematic of the typical two-room special acoustic test environment that is used for comprehensive speech audiometry. It can be used also for pure tone audiometry with older children and adults.

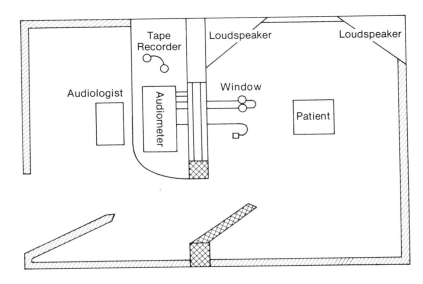

Speech Discrimination

Although the SRT offers an index of the degree of hearing loss for speech, it does not provide any information about the patient's ability to make distinctions among the various phonemic clues in our spoken language at conversational levels or at levels well above threshold. Consequently, numerous auditory speech discrimination tests have been developed for the purpose of assessing a patient's capability to *understand* conversational speech. The three most common types of tests involve the use of monosyllabic phonetically balanced word lists, monosyllabic multiple-choice word lists, and sentence tests. Considerable research has been conducted and reported on these different materials and used by clinicians throughout the world. The most popular tests consist of 25 or 50 phonetically balanced monosyllabic word lists.

The outcome of each of these tests is reported in percentage words correct. Table 8–2 summarizes a guideline for the interpretation of scores for a phonetically balanced monosyllabic word list, usually referred to as a PB list. The typical PB list contains 50 words, but many clinicians use 25 words or half lists. When this is done, the reliability of the test suffers, particularly in those cases in which the score is between 40 per cent and 90 per cent. That is, the fewer words used, the greater the test-retest variability. A 12 per cent difference from test to test is considered significant when 50 words are used. When 25 words are used, one must allow for a 24 per cent difference before assigning any significance to a change in discrimination.

All words in a speech discrimination test sample are usually presented at a fixed sensation level relative to the patient's speech reception threshold or pure tone average. This level will vary by clinician, but 30 to 40 dB above threshold (sensation level or SL) is most common. Many clinicians use the most comfortable level (MCL) for the presentation of speech discrimination material, especially if a patient cannot tolerate loud sound. This level is established by asking the patient to report his most comfortable loudness level while the clinician varies the intensity of speech. Other clinicians use several predetermined levels above threshold and obtain an articulation index or phonetically balanced–performance index (PB–PI) function or curve that usually ranges from poor speech discrimination to optimum performance at some level above threshold. Usually the speech discrimination scores will remain essentially constant, with increasing levels once the optimum score is obtained. If a score becomes significantly worse (20 per cent or more) with increasing levels, it is commonly referred to as a "rollover" phenomenon or function (Jerger 1970). The presence of rollover suggests a retrocochlear disorder (eighth nerve or brainstem). There is ample evidence in the literature that supports the fact that in a large number of patients with sensorineural hearing loss, the maximum speech discrimination score cannot be measured if the clinician uses only one sensation level as a routine. The exception, of course, is when the score is 92 per cent or 94 per cent or better at the chosen level. Clearly, if the score is less than this at a single level, the clinician cannot accurately predict the score if the test words were presented at another level. This evidence supports the use of more than one level for speech discrimination testing.

Speech discrimination tests are performed in a quiet, noncompetitive mode, as well as in the presence of a competing signal, such as speech, white noise, random noise, or some type of environmental noise. Patients invariably perform better or the same in quiet conditions, than in conditions in which there is competition. Whether or not the competitive signal is used in the speech discrimination test will depend upon the circumstances of the audiologic evaluation. The introduction of a competing message

Table 8–2. INTERPRETATION OF SPEECH DISCRIMINATION SCORES

Score (%)	Interpretation
90–100	Normal—no difficulty
80–89	Good—a little difficulty sometimes
60–79	Fair—noticeable difficulty sometimes
40–59	Poor—difficulty most of the time
<40	Very poor—much difficulty most of the time

will place greater stress on the patient's capacity to perform on a speech discrimination test. Competing message tests generally are more sensitive than noncompeting tests and thus are commonly used when attempting to establish a finer site of lesion for an auditory disorder, especially a lesion in the brainstem or at the cortical level. The use of competing message for patients with very poor discrimination in quiet (noncompeting) conditions is questionable. Usually in such instances, when the competition is introduced, the patient's ability to recognize the test words is so poor that the score is zero or close to nil. This type of testing offers little reward. Thus, competition is most valuable in cases in which the discrimination is fair to good. Under such circumstances, it is possible to observe the effect of a competing message on the patient's performance. Various primary signal-to-competition (or secondary) ratios (P/C or P/S) are employed ranging from a -10 to $+10$ dB. For example, a -10 P/S ratio means that the test words (P) are 10 dB more intense than the competition or secondary material (S).

Speech audiometry is one of the three components of the basic audiologic evaluation. It cannot be applied to a segment of the clinical population, such as very young children; patients with a serious speech, voice, or language disorder; patients who do not speak or understand the language spoken by the clinician; and other patients in whom spoken language presents a problem. In such cases, an important aspect of the audiologic evaluation is lost, even though modified versions of speech audiometry may be applied. Although speech audiometry has its limitations, it provides information about the functional efficiency of the patient's auditory system and, at the same time, may serve as a screening tool for identifying a finer site of lesion, e.g., cochlear versus eighth nerve or brainstem lesion.

IMPEDANCE AUDIOMETRY

The third popular component of a basic audiologic evaluation is impedance audiometry. This procedure is used to establish or confirm the type of hearing loss present as well as delineate the nature of a conductive component and to provide a clue to a possible eighth nerve or brainstem disorder. Impedance audiometry may be used in young children and other difficult-to-test patients to ascertain the audiometric configuration. This measurement was developed as a clinical technique during the late 1950s and 1960s in the Scandinavian countries. It found its way into the United States in the early 1970s. During the 1970s, it proved to be such a valuable clinical tool that it has taken its place as a fundamental procedure in a competent basic audiologic evaluation. In fact, in some clinical settings, impedance audiometry is the first procedure a patient undergoes because the result can usually predict the type and degree of hearing loss that will be found with pure tone audiometry. That is, a clinician can often predict the outcome of pure tone audiometry from the results of impedance audiometry and, as a consequence, save steps and time in routine pure tone measurements. Since impedance audiometry is an objective measure and pure tone audiometry is an inferential measure, impedance is a more dependable technique in cases in which there is some question of pure tone test validity.

According to Martin and Forbex, impedance audiometry is used routinely by an estimated 85 per cent of the practicing audiologists. This technique is especially useful in the evaluation of difficult-to-test populations, including very young children. It has been described for this purpose by Bluestone and associates as "the single most powerful tool at our disposal in the assessment of otitic disorders in children." This sensitive and objective clinical tool is used by audiologists to predict pure tone audiologic findings, identify the presence of middle ear effusion and facial nerve function, identify functional hearing loss, and assist in the diagnosis of the site of the auditory lesion.

Impedance audiometry is based on physical acoustic principles. When a sound wave (pure tone) strokes the eardrum, a portion of the signal is transmitted through the middle ear to the cochlea, whereas the remaining portion is reflected back into the ear canal. The reflective energy forms a wave traveling in an outward direction, whose phase and amplitude is dependent upon the opposition encountered at the tympanic membrane. The energy of the reflected wave is greatest when the middle ear system is stiff or immobile, as in the case of certain middle ear disorders. On the other hand, when the air pressure on both sides of the eardrum with no middle ear disorder is essentially equal, or when the ossicular chain is disarticulated, consid-

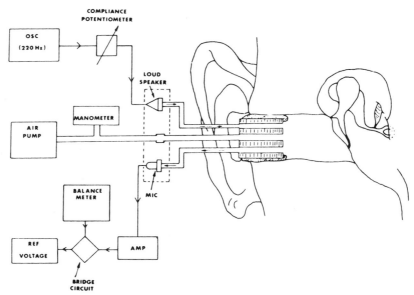

Figure 8–23. Schematic representation of an electroacoustic impedance meter with probe tip inserted into an ear canal. This unit consists of an oscillator that produces a probe tone (220 Hz), an air pressure monometer, and a microphone that compares the sound pressure in the ear canal with a reference sound pressure.

erably less sound energy will be reflected back into the ear canal. Thus, a greater portion of the sound wave will be absorbed by the eardrum and middle ear. Impedance audiometry involves the measurement of a sound wave introduced to a hermetically sealed ear canal. This measurement is conducted while a control stimulus is introduced to the ear. The stimulus is designed to cause changes in the status of the eardrum or contraction of the middle ear muscles.

Figure 8–23 is a schematic of a typical acoustic impedance measuring instrument. A probe tip containing three small holes is sealed into the ear canal. Through one port, a low-frequency "probe tone" (usually 220 Hz) is delivered into the ear canal at about 90 dB SPL. Another port leads to a sensitive microphone that senses the SPL of the probe tone. The third port leads from an air pump, which allows the air pressure, measured in millimeters of water pressure, to be varied in the sealed ear canal. The measuring network of the impedance audiometer quantifies changes in the probe tone while the air pressure is varied in the ear canal or while the stapedial muscle reflex is elicited. Figure 8–24 is an illustration of a modern impedance audiometer.

Basic Impedance Test Battery

There are three measurements involved in basic impedance audiometry: tympanometry, stapedial reflex threshold, and stapedial reflex decay measurement. The patient's ear canal must be reasonably free of debris and cerumen, and the eardrum must be intact in order for the physician to carry out these procedures.

Tympanometry. Tympanometry involves the simultaneous tracking of a probe pure tone and variation in air pressure in a sealed ear canal. The air pressure variation typically covers a range of from +200 mm H_2O to −300 or −400 mm H_2O. When the eardrum reaches its most compliant state during this change in air pressure, the system will measure the maximum decrease in the level of the probe tone. A normal tympanogram is shown in Figure 8–25. Those who elect to categorize tympanograms refer to this tracing as a type A. Note that the increase in compliance is indicated by an upward excursion of the tracing, reaching its maximum at approximately 0 mm H_2O. At this point, the patient should experience an increase in the loudness of the probe tone. Figure 8–26 shows a tympanogram for

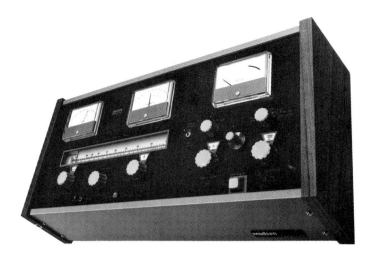

Figure 8–24. Impedance audiometer. (Madsen Model 2072D). (Courtesy of Madsen Electronics, Oakville, Ontario.)

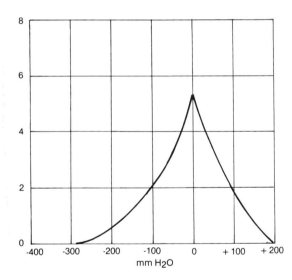

Figure 8–25. Typical normal tympanogram showing a pressure/compliance curve obtained by changing air pressure in millimeters of water from +200 to −300 in a sealed ear canal. This curve is commonly referred to as type A.

Figure 8–26. A typical "flat" tympanogram that shows an absence of a pressure/compliance peak across a range from +200 mm H_2O to −400 mm H_2O. This is commonly referred to as a type B tympanogram. This tympanogram indicates gross middle ear effusion or massive ossicular fixation.

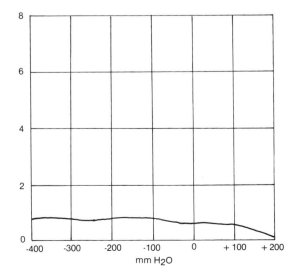

a patient with otitis media with effusion. Note the absence of change in compliance as the air pressure is changed. This is often referred to as a type B tracing. Figure 8–27 is a typical example of ossicular discontinuity. Note the extreme increase in compli-

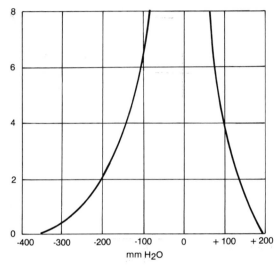

Figure 8–27. A typical high compliance tympanogram that suggests an ossicular discontinuity in the presence of a conductive hearing loss. Some patients with normal hearing will manifest high compliance because of a very flaccid drum.

ance as the air pressure in the ear canal passes through zero ambient or atmospheric pressure. Some label this a type A_D tracing. Figure 8–28 shows a maximum pressure/compliance point in the negative pressure zone (-250 mm H_2O), which indicates negative pressure in the middle ear. Type C is the label attached to this type of measurement. This measurement suggests a middle ear effusion that is ensuing or in remission. At least, a type C tympanogram indicates a malfunctioning eustachian tube.

Normal tympanogram configuration is found in normal individuals, patients with pure sensorineural hearing loss, and those with conductive losses due to stapedial fixation (e.g., otosclerosis). Simple fixation of the stapedial footplate seems to have little effect on reducing the compliance of the eardrum during changes in air pressure. A flat tympanogram (type B) or negative peak pressure tympanograms (type C) are customary in patients with middle ear effusion, middle ear tissue mass, or massive ossicular fixation. A tympanogram with the maximum pressure/compliance point in the negative range (greater than 150 mm H_2O) that is peaked rather than rounded (type C) indicates insufficient eustachian tube function, with a high probability of a dry middle ear cleft. Finally, a highly compliant eardrum

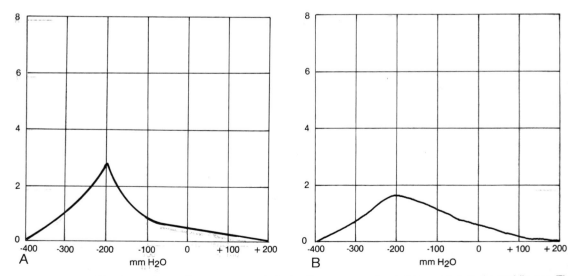

Figure 8–28. A, This form of type C tympanogram indicates the presence of negative pressure in the middle ear. The maximum pressure/compliance peak occurs in the -200 mm H_2O region. This is indicative of a middle ear with no effusion. B, This type C tympanogram with a rounded maximum/pressure/compliance peak in a negative region is indicative of some middle ear effusion with negative middle ear pressure.

(type D) in the presence of a significant conductive hearing loss strongly suggests disruption of the ossicular chain.

Acoustic Reflex Threshold. It is well accepted today that intense sound will elicit the stapedial acoustic reflex. Stated differently, the acoustic reflex is probably a loudness-mediated phenomenon. This action is normally bilateral, even when the intense sound is delivered to just one ear. This physiologic activity facilitates the convenient measure of the acoustic stapedial reflex threshold using pure tones. Although the average reflex threshold varies slightly by frequency, it occurs within a range of 75 to 95 dB HL in most normal ears. When an acoustic reflex is measured by stimulating the ear opposite the probe tip, it is referred to as a contralateral or crossed acoustic reflex. When a reflex is elicited by stimulating the ear containing the probe tip, it is called an ipsilateral or uncrossed acoustic reflex. The use of both crossed and uncrossed acoustic reflexes offers more clinical flexibility and a higher level of sophistication for the establishment of differential diagnostic information for the site of an auditory lesion.

The acoustic reflex threshold can be obtained in patients with a pure sensorineural hearing loss if the loss is not too severe (greater than or equal to 80 dB HL). According to Jerger, the probability of eliciting the acoustic reflex in patients with a greater than 80-dB HL decreases markedly because of the degree of loss in auditory sensitivity. Consequently, acoustic reflex thresholds should be obtainable for the majority of patients with a sensorineural hearing loss. Furthermore, the acoustic reflex threshold for patients with a mild or moderate hearing loss will be at about the same hearing level as that for people with normal hearing. Since the most tenable explanation for mediation of the acoustic reflex is the loudness of a sound, this observation supports the use of the acoustic reflex as a loudness recruitment test. In fact, this was the initial intent for the clinical use of the acoustic reflex test (Metz, 1946). Today, there are numerous other applications for the acoustic reflex threshold test, but in the basic audiologic evaluation, it is used primarily to establish the presence of a pure sensorineural hearing loss due to a cochlear lesion. Conversely, it is used, along with tympanometry, to confirm the presence of a conductive lesion, since it is absent in nearly all conductive hearing losses. If the reflex is absent or elevated out of proportion to the degree of hearing loss in a patient with a pure sensorineural loss, one must suspect a retrocochlear disorder.

Acoustic Reflex Decay. The third measure in the impedance test battery is the acoustic reflex decay test. This measurement immediately follows determination of the stapedial reflex threshold. A pure tone is presented at a level 10 dB above the acoustic reflex threshold for a period of 10 seconds. The initial magnitude of the reflex is used as the full or whole life of the reflex. Abnormal reflex decay occurs if the magnitude of the reflex diminishes to one half of or less than its full life within 10 seconds. Figure 8–29 shows examples of no reflex decay and of abnormal decay. This measure is limited to 500 or 1000 Hz because by this criteria, people with normal hearing or a cochlear lesion will show reflex decay for frequencies above 1000 Hz. The presence of abnormal reflex decay is indicative of an eighth nerve or brainstem disorder.

Impedance audiometry, in conjunction with pure tone and speech audiometry, has greatly strengthened the value of the basic audiologic evaluation. It is not a substitute for pure tone and speech audiometry. Instead, it provides additional information about the status and functioning of the auditory system that pure tone and speech audiometry cannot provide. Its value in the basic audiologic evaluation is well expressed by Jerger: "We frankly wonder how we ever got along without it."

Even though impedance audiometry is a sensitive, objective clinical tool that offers

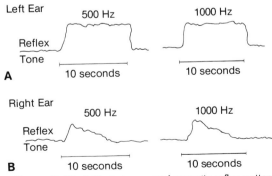

Figure 8–29. A illustrates normal acoustic reflex pattern for a 10-second pure tone stimuli presented 10 dB above (sensation level) the acoustic reflex threshold. B shows an acoustic reflex pattern that decreases or decays in less than 10 seconds to at least one half of the initial magnitude of the reflex that was present on introduction of the eliciting stimulus.

valuable information on a variety of questions about the status of the auditory mechanism, it does have some limitations in the basic audiologic evaluation. Probably one of the biggest problems we encounter using impedance audiometry is the inability to obtain an airtight seal in some ear canals. It seems that this problem occurs in patients for whom we must rely heavily on impedance audiometry for some basic information, e.g., very young children and patients with early retrocochlear symptoms or questionable mixed losses. There is a need to have a probe tip available that will invariably offer a seal, even in the most distorted ear canals. Thus, it is recommended that physicians with a busy clinical practice have a wide variety of ear canal sealing devices. Cerumen can be a problem in clinics in which medical personnel are inaccessible. Obviously, the ear canal must be reasonably clean to allow for impedance audiometry. Tympanic membrane perforations can be identified by impedance audiometry. The tympanogram will be flat and the volume measured will be high in the case of a perforation with no eustachian tube function. Even a small perforation may preclude a valid impedance measure. The tympanogram will be flat and the volume measured will be high. Thus, patients with tympanostomy tubes cannot be tested except to determine the patency of the tube. There is still the need for more research on the interpretation of tympanograms as they relate to the presence or absence of middle ear effusion.

Instrumentation for impedance audiometry is critical for accurate measurements. For the most part, commercial instruments are of good quality, but must be checked frequently for accuracy. The American National Standards Institute has recently promulgated specifications for impedance instruments, which should help to maintain more consistent standards of design and construction in the industry.

Examples of Results From Basic Audiologic Evaluations

This section contains some typical examples of results obtained from pure tone, speech, and impedance audiometry. Each example is accompanied by a brief explanation of the test results.

Case number 1 (Fig. 8–30) is a 12-year-old patient with bilateral serous otitis media. In

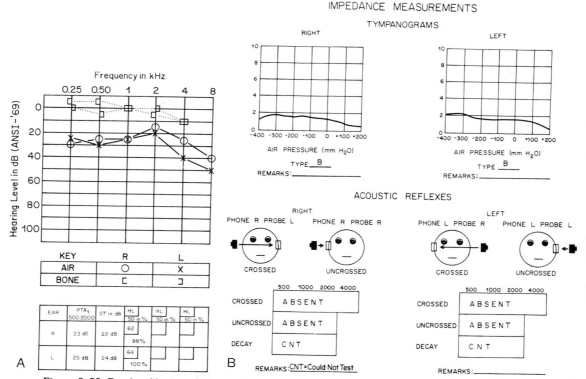

Figure 8–30. Results of basic audiologic evaluation of a 12-year-old patient with bilateral serous otitis media.

such a case, a mild loss in sensitivity, as evidenced by the pure tone air-conduction thresholds and SRT, is usually seen. There is an air-bone gap, and speech discrimination is excellent. The tympanograms are essentially flat (type B), and the acoustic reflex is absent in both ears.

Case number 2 (Fig. 8–31) is a 30-year-old patient with bilateral otosclerosis. The audiogram shows a moderate, bilaterally symmetric conductive hearing loss with a jagged audiometric configuration, which is typical in such cases. The speech thresholds agree well with the pure tone averages, and speech discrimination is excellent, as is the case in essentially all pure conductive hearing losses. The tympanograms are normal (type A) in shape, but with somewhat reduced compliance, and the acoustic reflex is absent for both ears.

Case number 3 (Fig. 8–32) is a 25-year-old patient with a moderate, left unilateral conductive hearing loss due to interruption of the ossicular chain. In such cases, a maximum conductive loss of 60- to 70-dB HL, good agreement between SRT and pure tone average, and excellent speech discrimination are often seen. The tympanogram for the good ear is normal (type A_D). The crossed

acoustic reflex is absent for both ears, and the uncrossed is absent in the impaired ear, but present and normal in the good ear.

Case number 4 (Fig. 8–33) is a 76-year-old patient with a hearing loss diagnosed as presbycusis. The audiogram shows a mild-to-moderate, bilaterally symmetric pure sensorineural hearing loss with a gradually falling audiometric configuration. Speech thresholds agree reasonably well with the pure tone averages, and the patient's discrimination for speech is fair. Many elderly patients who report an insidious onset of hearing loss manifest this type of audiometric picture. Speech discrimination is often impaired, but not always. Impedance audiometry shows normal tympanograms; the acoustic reflex is in the normal range, with no reflex decay.

Case number 5 (Fig. 8–34) is a 42-year-old patient with Meniere's syndrome. Here a moderate right unilateral sensorineural hearing loss with a gradually rising audiometric configuration, peaking at 2000 Hz and falling off at 8000 Hz, is seen. The SRT agrees with the pure tone average. Speech discrimination is quite poor, but there is no rollover at high presentation levels. Tympanograms are normal (type A) for both ears, and the acous-

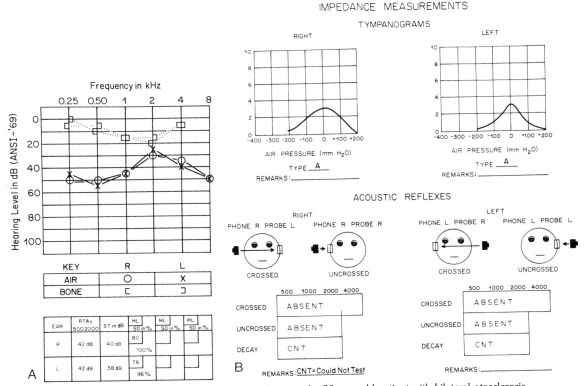

Figure 8–31. Results of basic audiologic evaluation of a 30-year-old patient with bilateral otosclerosis.

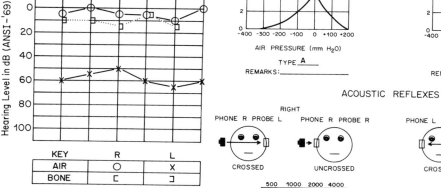

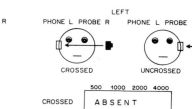

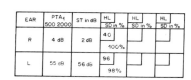

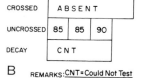

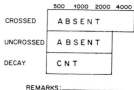

Figure 8–32. Results of basic audiologic evaluation of a 25-year-old patient with a moderate unilateral conductive hearing loss in the left ear caused by interruption of the ossicular chain.

Figure 8–33. Results of basic audiologic evaluation of a 76-year-old patient with a hearing loss diagnosed as presbycusis.

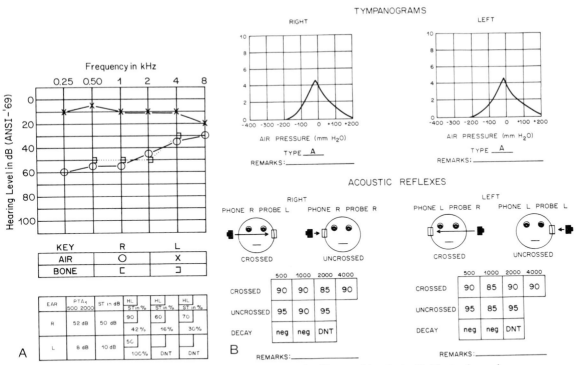

Figure 8–34. Results of basic audiologic evaluation of a 42-year-old patient with Meniere's syndrome.

tic reflex thresholds are within normal range bilaterally. The reduced sensation level for the acoustic reflexes in the impaired ear indicates loudness recruitment, which is typical in cochlear lesions. That is, the acoustic reflex thresholds occur at the same hearing level in the impaired ear as in the normal hearing ear. Finally, there is no reflex decay. These results are typical of a cochlear disorder.

Case number 6 (Fig. 8–35) is a 50-year-old patient with a hearing loss resulting from a meningioma in the left ear. The audiogram shows a bilateral sensorineural hearing loss that is greater in the left ear, with an asymmetric audiometric configuration. The speech threshold agrees with the pure tone averages and speech discrimination is good in the right ear but fair-to-poor in the left, with marked rollover at high presentation levels. Poor speech discrimination is a common finding in patients with eighth nerve disorder. Tympanometry further confirms a pure sensorineural hearing loss with normal bilateral tympanograms. Crossed and uncrossed acoustic reflexes are absent for the left ear but are present for the right. Acoustic

reflexes are often absent in eighth nerve lesions when the hearing loss is mild or moderate in degree. Thus, in such cases it is impossible to conduct the acoustic reflex decay test. An eighth nerve lesion should be suspected for all patients with an asymmetric pure sensorineural hearing loss until proven otherwise.

Case number 7 (Fig. 8–36) is a 24-year-old patient with a sudden bilateral hearing loss due to a blow to the head. The pure tone audiogram shows a moderate bilaterally symmetric mixed hearing loss with a trough-shaped audiometric configuration. The speech thresholds are 20 to 26 dB better than the pure tone average, and speech discrimination is excellent at levels approximating the pure tone averages. Tympanograms are normal (type A), which is unusual in mixed losses unless they are caused by stapedial fixation, but the acoustic reflex thresholds are present and within the normal range, which contraindicates a conductive component. This finding definitely rules out a mixed loss. These overall findings indicate a functional hearing loss. The discrepancy between the SRT and pure tone averages,

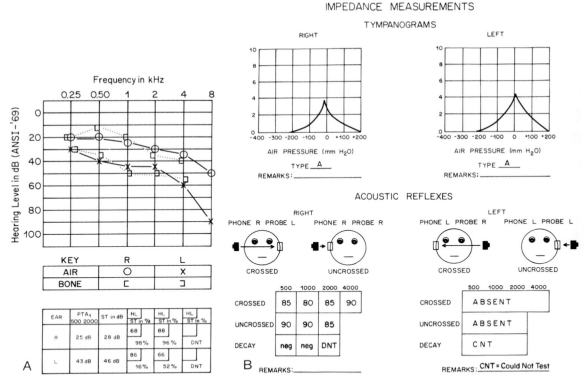

Figure 8–35. Results of basic audiologic evaluation of a 50-year-old patient with hearing loss from a left meningioma.

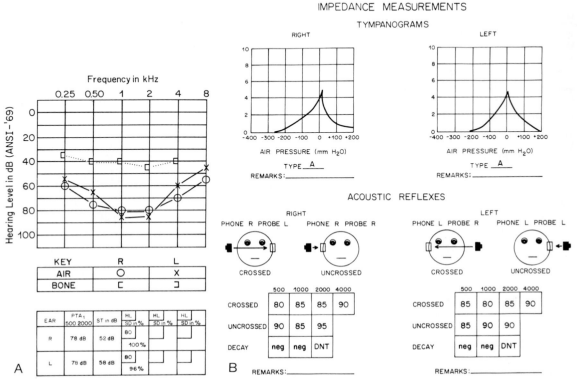

Figure 8–36. Results of basic audiologic evaluation of a 24-year-old patient with a sudden bilateral hearing loss as a result of a blow to the head.

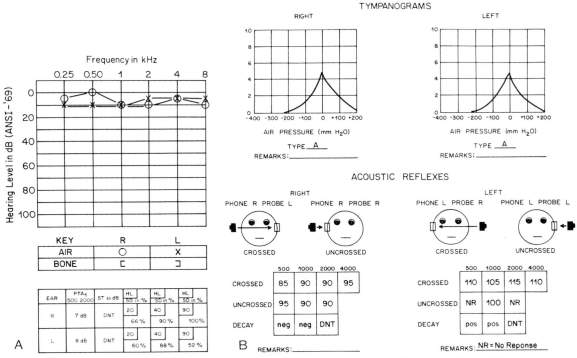

Figure 8–37. Results of basic audiologic evaluation of a 38-year-old patient with slight unsteadiness, left tinnitus, and a muffled sensation in the left ear.

the good discrimination at pure tone threshold levels, and the normal impedance all point toward a functional disorder.

Case number 8 (Fig. 8–37) is a 38-year-old patient who complains of a slight unsteadiness, left tinnitus, and a muffled sensation in the left ear. The pure tone audiogram is normal; therefore it was unnecessary to determine speech thresholds. However, there is a significant rollover effect for speech discrimination in the left ear. Impedance measurements yield normal tympanograms for both ears, but the crossed and uncrossed acoustic reflex thresholds for the left ear are elevated. There is marked reflex decay of the left ear. An early eighth nerve or low brainstem disorder must be suspected in this patient until proven otherwise.

If a handicapping hearing loss persists after the cause of a hearing loss is determined and maximum medical or surgical remediation has been carried out, use of a hearing aid should be considered. In some patients, especially children, with a persistent conductive or mixed hearing loss that is slow in responding to medical or surgical intervention, use of a hearing aid may be appropriate during treatment. The next section of this chapter provides a comprehensive overview of the hearing aid, which is the logical alternative in the remedial management of patients with irreversible hearing loss.

Amplification for the Hearing Impaired

There are about 15 million people in the United States who probably could benefit from an appropriately fitted amplification device. However, less than half this number have hearing aids. One of the reasons why more people do not use amplification is because of misinformation about hearing aids by the public as well as the medical profession. Consequently, patients are often steered away from amplification by their physician or avoid investigating a hearing aid because of a preconceived notion that one will not help. Another problem is that many people consult a dispenser who lacks adequate training and credentials in hearing-aid technology, fitting, and auditory rehabilitation. A credentialed (certified, registered, licensed) audiologist is the most likely professional to consult for hearing-aid rehabilitation.

A hearing aid is quite basic in design, but because of its size and the hard use that most receive, it is a highly technical device. Every hearing aid contains four basic components, which are illustrated in Figure 8–38. First, a microphone receives sound and converts it into an electrical signal. Second, an amplifier increases the amplitude of the electrical signal. The amplifier requires energy from a power source, which is a small battery. A miniature loudspeaker, called an earphone or receiver, completes the basic system. This component converts the amplified electrical signals back into acoustic energy or sound and delivers it into the ear. All hearing aids, regardless of size or appearance, are composed of these four components.

The four types of hearing aids available today are shown in Figure 8–39. Body aids are worn in a harness, in a shirt pocket, or pinned to underclothing. This type of aid is used by people with a severe degree of hearing loss or by those with poor manual dexterity, who need large visible controls in order to operate the instrument. The other three types of aids are worn on the head. The postauricular type of aid is the most popular; the in-the-ear type of aid is next in popularity, with the eyeglass and body aids a low third and fourth in order of use.

Determination of those who can benefit from a hearing aid is one of the most misunderstood aspects concerning the treatment of the hearing impaired. Advances in miniature electronic technology make it possible to provide effective amplification for people with virtually all types and degrees of hearing impairment. Probably the most unfortunate myth about hearing aids is that patients with "nerve deafness" cannot use amplification. This is totally incorrect. In fact, the vast majority of hearing aid users today have a sensorineural or mixed-type hearing loss. Sophisticated techniques now make it possible to fit patients with sensorineural hearing loss, unilateral loss, high-frequency loss, severe hearing impairment, and mild loss and even those with reduced tolerance for loud sounds. Of course, some patients are much more difficult to rehabilitate than others, and some simply cannot adjust to and use amplification. However, under competent professional management, the number of failures today is extremely small.

Using an audiogram to determine who can and who cannot benefit from a hearing aid can be misleading and inaccurate. Probably the simplest approach to determining if a patient is a candidate for a hearing aid is to ask two questions: (1) Do you have trouble hearing in your daily life activities? and (2) Do you want to improve your hearing? If the answers to both of these questions are affirmative, the patient automatically becomes a candidate for a hearing aid. Although this approach gets directly to the point in most cases, it is by no means foolproof. Some patients, particularly in the geriatric population, will deny hearing loss and must be urged to investigate the use of an aid. Other patients will admit to a hearing loss but will refuse to wear an aid. Many of these patients have been discouraged by a hearing-impaired friend who has had an unfortunate experience with amplification. In any event, the patient should be referred to a competent audiologist who knows hearing aids and preferably also dispenses aids. Such practice is more likely to ensure appropriate and optimal amplification, resulting in patient satisfaction.

If the audiologist determines that amplification may help the patient's communicative problem, the selection of either one or two (binaural) appropriate hearing aids is warranted. Many clinicians refer to this as the preselection process, which as a result of the vast array of options currently available for wearable amplification is often rather complex. The objective is to provide the patient with amplification that will offer optimal hearing efficiency within the limitations imposed by the damage to the patient's auditory system. The following is a list of the major options or variables that

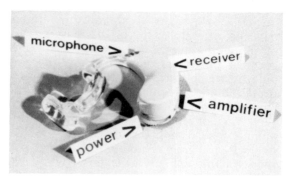

Figure 8–38. Basic components of a hearing aid. All hearing aids, regardless of their appearance, contain these four components.

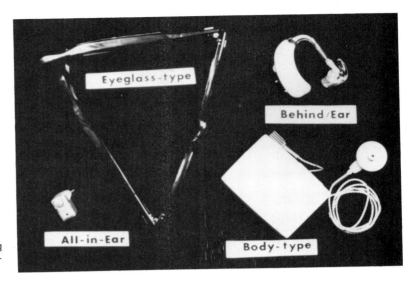

Figure 8–39. Four types of hearing aids: body, postauricular (behind-the-ear), eyeglass, and in-the-ear.

need to be considered when selecting a hearing aid for a patient:

Type of aid
  Body, postauricular, eyeglass, in-the-ear
Mode of amplification
  Monaural direct to right or left ear; binaural; monaural indirect
  (CROS) to right or left ear; monaural indirect and monaural direct
  (BI-CROS or MULTI-CROS)
Gain
Frequency response
Saturation sound pressure level or maximum power output
Type of output limiting
Directional or omni-directional microphone
Coupling
  Full-open canal, vented, occluded
Hearing aid–tinnitus masker combination

Recognizing that differences exist between various makes and models of hearing aids, as well as between the different types of hearing impairment, it is understandable that patients vary in their needs for amplification. Thus, numerous procedures have been proposed over the past 30 years that provide a basis upon which a patient can be advised to procure a particular hearing aid. Differences of opinion have always existed among audiologists regarding the best way to select a hearing aid for a patient. Clinicians tend to adopt a procedure that seems to work well for them and with which they are comfortable.

Generally speaking, the procedure used to select a hearing aid for a patient will fall into one of three categories or any combination of the three: (1) catalogue selection based on matching electroacoustic characteristics to the patient's hearing loss, (2) trial and error listening to one or more aids by the patient, and (3) some "objective" comparative procedure involving the conduct of tests while the patient is wearing one or more hearing aids. There are three assumptions concerning hearing aids that most audiologists recognize, even though there may not be clinical procedures to support all of them: They are the following: (1) Hearing aids vary in the way that they help people understand speech, (2) the relative effectiveness of various hearing aids differs from one patient to the next, and (3) real differences in patient performance with various hearing aids can be measured by some type of reliable test. It is this third assumption that results in most of the controversy among clinicians that was mentioned earlier. There is a real need for a reliable objective technique that will allow for the verification of hearing-aid performance while the aid is being worn by the patient. Such a technique is certain to be available within the foreseeable future.

Regardless of the specific procedure used to select a hearing aid for a patient, the main objectives of most audiologists engaged in hearing-aid selection can be summarized as follows: (1) to assess the patient's need for amplification, (2) to estimate how well the patient will function with an amplifying stem, and (3) to determine the electroacoustic and acoustic characteristics needed for effective amplification for a specific patient. At the conclusion of this stage of the process, the patient is most likely to be advised to do one of the following:

1. Retain the present hearing aid because it is functioning well and providing optimal benefit.

2. Retain the present hearing aid, but with some specific modifications.

3. Purchase a new aid according to specific characteristics.

4. Avoid use of a hearing aid at the present time and return for re-evaluation in 1 year or sooner if hearing should become worse.

After a hearing aid is selected, it is important to maintain periodic contact with the patient because virtually all new users go through an adjustment period. Many times it is necessary for the audiologist to change the gain, frequency response, or maximum output of the aid to better meet the communicative and comfort needs of the patient. One purpose of return visits with the new aid is to enable the physician to assess the patient's performance and experiences. Another objective is to offer appropriate orientation and counseling to ensure effective adjustment to amplification and use of the hearing aid. It is critically important that the patient have the intelligence and the skill to regulate the volume control and switches, insert and remove the earmold and battery, and control other important aspects of the hearing aid and earmold. Inserting, using, and caring for a hearing aid are considerably more complex than using contact lenses. To complicate matters even more, a hearing aid is less likely to compensate as effectively for a hearing impairment as contact lenses do for a visual deficit. Thus, the patient must be tolerant, educable, and, indeed, patient. Under competent professional guidance and supervision, the vast majority of patients should turn into satisfied hearing-aid users. Encouragement and support by the physician is quite beneficial. If a patient reports that he could not adjust to a hearing aid, it may be the result of his own incapacities or it may be that he was under poor professional management. Simply because a patient reports that he has not benefitted from a hearing aid is no reason to assume that a hearing aid will not help him.

A thorough follow-up service is as important to the total program of hearing-aid selection as the hearing-aid selection itself. The problem, of course, is getting the patient to return after procuring the aid, especially if it is dispensed in a location other than that of the audiologic and otologic care. It is the opinion of an ever-increasing number of audiologists that the clinician is responsible for dispensing hearing aids as part of comprehensive hearing health care. Such total services are now available to the hearing impaired throughout the United States. The hearing impaired patient should be advised to seek professional care at a place in which audiologic care and hearing-aid dispensing are all offered.

BIBLIOGRAPHY

Bluestone, C. D., Beery, Q. C., and Paradise, J. L.: Audiometry and Tympanometry in relation to middle ear effusions in children. Laryngoscope 83:594–604, 1973.

Carhart, R.: Atypical audiometric configurations associated with otosclerosis. Ann Otol Rhinol Laryngol 71:744–758, 1962.

Harford, E. R.: Hearing aid amplification for adults. In Schwartz, D., and Bess, F. (eds.): Monographs in Contemporary Audiology. Minneapolis, Maico Hearing Instruments, 1979.

Jerger, J.: Clinical experience with impedance audiometry. Arch Otolaryngol 92, 311–324, 1970.

Jerger, J.: Modern Developments in Audiology, 2nd ed. New York, Academic Press, 1973.

Jerger, J., and Jerger, S.: Diagnostic audiology. In Tower, D. (ed.): The Nervous System. Vol. 3. New York, Raven Press, 1975, 199–205.

Jerger, J., and Jerger, S.: Clinical validity of central auditory tests. Scand. Audiol. 4, 147.

Jerger, J., and Northern, J. L.: Clinical Impedance Audiometry. Acton, Mass, American Electromedics Corp., 1980.

Jerger, S., and Jerger, J.: Auditory Disorders. Boston, Little, Brown and Co., 1981.

Katz, J.: Handbook of Clinical Audiology. 2nd ed. Baltimore, Williams and Wilkins Co., 1978.

Martin, F. N., and Forbis, N. K.: The present status of audiometric practice. ASHA. 20:531–541, 1978.

Metz, O.: The acoustic impedance measured on normal and pathological ears. Acta Otolaryngol Suppl. 63, 1254–1264, 1946.

Rintelmann, W.: Hearing Assessment Baltimore, University Park Press, 1979.

David W. Johnson

9

SCREENING, SEARCH, AND IDENTIFICATION: STRATEGIES FOR REFERRAL

Auditory screening is a system for the identification of an auditory pathologic condition before it becomes obvious. A discussion of "screening" must begin with a basic understanding of "role." The health provider must understand the purpose of the setting in which health care is rendered. It is that sense of purpose that ultimately defines the type of screening.

Screening may be different in different settings because purposes vary. Subpopulations within the broader patient clientele may have specific needs that may have to be addressed without involving all patients in a screening procedure. Targeting the needs of a population is necessary if an appropriate screening procedure for hearing problems is to be established.

From the outset, the otolaryngologist needs to see screening as an avenue for using others to identify hearing loss and direct patients with hearing health care needs into the specialty practice. Indirectly, the screening program may use nonphysician personnel, thereby freeing the primary practitioner as well as the otolaryngologist for more cost-effective use of time.

Goal of Hearing Screening

Essentially, the goal of screening of hearing is identification of ear disease that can be managed medically, surgically, or through rehabilitation. Rehabilitation can be achieved through management of patients' respective listening environments or through amplification. This goal incorporates the control of active disease and the maximization of communicative adequacy for daily living.

Communicative adequacy is especially important (see Table 8–1). The very young (preschool and early school age) patient must have sufficient hearing to adequately develop speech, language, and social skills in order to function well in a hearing society. At the other end of the age spectrum, the geriatric patient must have sufficient hearing to be comfortable in changing social environments in which new people and social interactions are encountered. These may include senior citizen activity centers, retirement communities, or nursing homes. The geriatric patient may need help with hearing just to maintain any quality of life. Auditory needs include sufficient hearing for religious services or other group activities in which understanding the spoken voice is so crucial to happiness. Between these two age spectrums are people who may have hearing problems that will impact on family relationships, recreational activities, and employment.

If hearing function cannot be brought into an acceptable range through physician intervention alone, medical and surgical management of ear disease must be supported by auditory rehabilitation. Unfortunately, pure tone acuity at several frequencies has been

153

interpreted as the measure of social adequacy by some in the otolaryngologic community. Therefore, in dealing with screening data, it is necessary to be problem-oriented rather than audiogram-oriented. By implication, it is unconscionable to develop a screening program, get the patient referred, see the patient, and then not deal with the problem that the patient brings to the physician. The otolaryngologist may maintain that "hearing loss is a symptom of disease," but a hearing problem is a "hearing" problem, which needs a "hearing" answer when medical and surgical management have been exhausted or ruled out.

Target Population of Hearing Screening

Who should be screened? The answer to this question is complex because one obviously does not want to screen too many "normals" or patients who have no hearing problem. On the other hand, one does not want to overlook an excessive number of patients suffering from hearing loss. Several strategies for determining target population should be considered, depending on the otolaryngologist and the setting of practice. Which strategy is utilized depends upon the screening personnel available, the methodology of the screening, and the patient population to be screened.

AGE-BASED STRATEGY

Children with hearing disorders suffer psychologically and educationally. Parents and educators frequently complain that hearing-impaired youngsters are not identified at an early enough age to provide early stimulation of speech and language. The cause of the hearing loss is not the crucial issue for parents and teachers. What is crucial is the psychosocial detriment and loss of education input time. It is, therefore, proper to provide auditory screening for all children, particularly when there are questions about whether speech and language maturation are normal.

On occasion, there may be a conflict of ideas concerning the medical management of children with fluctuating hearing loss. Although some primary practitioners may control active infection with medication, middle ear effusion may persist and induce speech and language delay in certain youngsters. The screening programs that are developed for children must take into consideration potential physician management issues. Physician consensus as to treatment alternatives may need to be specified at the time screening programs are implemented, particularly when assisting the primary health care provider with screening criteria for referral to the otolaryngology practice.

On the other end of the age spectrum, presbycusis is a fact of life in our society and relates both to a lifetime of environmental noise exposure and to tissue maturation and biochemical changes occurring in the aging process. Hearing loss may also begin at any age from disease or trauma. Hearing difficulties may begin in midlife when occupational noise exposure has been excessive. It is not so important to know specifically what age- and sex-adjusted presbycusis values are as it is to recognize that hearing loss increases as we age. Regardless of history, by age 60, significant numbers of people will manifest hearing problems.

Adults do not frequently complain about hearing problems, particularly when the onset of hearing loss has been gradual or buried sometime in the past. One is only too familiar with the individual whose ear canals are fully occluded with cerumen, which was discovered only by "accident" through a screening or when the patient presented for other health care concerns. Similarly, it may take repeated family suggestions for several years to bring an individual in to "get the wax out of my ears." Unfortunately, the patient often has clear external auditory canals and a more serious cause for the hearing loss. The hearing loss may be due to additive factors, such as large tympanic membrane perforations and presbycusis. The relatively mild hearing loss from the initial malady may not have affected the patient's everyday life at first, but the aging process and its effects on the inner ear brought hearing deterioration to the point at which the patient recognized the hearing problems. Routine screening, therefore, is suggested for those over 55 years of age and especially when family or friends suspect a hearing problem.

HIGH-RISK-BASED STRATEGY

A number of health care problems that are not specifically hearing-related have an impact on hearing function. Congenital factors

(Table 9–1), birth trauma, bacterial infections, viral infections, ototoxic drugs (Table 9–2), head trauma, and nose exposure may all potentially adversely affect hearing. Hereditary and biochemical factors associated with hearing problems may also predispose some individuals to hearing loss, and when such factors exist, it is appropriate to provide screening. Patients with known metabolic disease should also be screened for hearing loss or referred directly for baseline audiometrics prior to the implementation of treatment for the primary disease condition. Patients who are admitted to intensive care units, particularly newborns, should be screened.

COMMUNICATION-ADEQUACY STRATEGY

The ability to hear, listen, and understand are crucial for normal life. We live in a society in which the auditory modality is the primary information channel for so many things, such as doorbells, telephones, radio, motion pictures, television, and emergency alerting from car horns, ambulance sirens, and civil defense sirens. Hearing is also important for our interpersonal relationships.

ENVIRONMENT-BASED STRATEGY

People who have exposure to high levels of steady-state or impact noise in their daily lives may experience hearing loss. Ambulance drivers, police, truck drivers, assembly line workers, punch press operators, heavy equipment operators, miners, loggers, musicians, and even secretaries with noisy typewriters may be susceptible to noise-related health problems. Irritability, high blood pressure, fatigue, and temporary auditory threshold shift are not uncommon complaints when high levels of background noise are present in the work environs. The Occupational Safety and Health Administration has become more active in noise-related workplace problems. Workmen's compensation has been provided to those with noise-induced hearing loss. Companies have increasingly sought to avoid potential litigation by controlling noise exposure and by monitoring the hearing of those exposed to noise on a regular basis. If there are average noise levels in excess of 85 dB in the daily environment of a patient, appropriate

screening of that patient's hearing on a regular basis is suggested. Screening of hearing may be appropriate when there is suspicion of high levels of noise exposure, as, for example, when the patient complains that he has to raise his voice to be heard at work or whose hearing is worse in the evening after work than in the morning before work. Otologic referral is suggested if a baseline audiogram demonstrates an average hearing level at 0.5, 1, 2, and 3 kHz worse than 25 dB in either ear or a difference between ears of more than 15 dB at 0.5, 1, 2, kHz or more than 30 dB at 3, 4, and 6 kHz. Otologic referral is also suggested if there is a deterioration of hearing in either ear of more than 15 dB at 0.5, 1, and 2 kHz or more than 30 dB at 3, 4, and 6 kHz on periodic audiograms. Any patient with a history of otalgia, otorrhea, vertigo, severe tinnitus, or fluctuating or rapidly progressive hearing loss also deserves otologic referral.

CLINIC-BASED OR INSTITUTION-BASED STRATEGY

The nature of some kinds of practice requires regular monitoring of hearing for health care. A clinic designed to deal with children exclusively, an institution in which the mentally retarded are housed, and an industrial clinic serving people who are regularly exposed to noise are examples of such facilities. Appropriate screening of hearing is needed at any clinic or institution that sees a population in whom especially good hearing function is needed or in whom hearing problems are likely to occur at high incidence levels. Certainly the most common example of this type of screening procedure is the screening of hearing in public schools, which is done in many school districts. Routine screening may also take place in hospital outpatient departments as part of chronic dialysis programs.

Setting

Screening can be performed in a variety of places. The discussion that follows serves as a summary for screening in different settings.

THE FREE-STANDING INDIVIDUAL OTOLARYNGOLOGIC PRACTICE

The small private practice may have little need of the variety of screening programs
Text continued on page 165

Table 9–1. DISORDERS THAT MAY BE ASSOCIATED WITH HEARING LOSS*

Congenital Sensorineural Hearing Loss

Craniofacial and Skeletal Disorders

Klippel-Feil syndrome	Recessive or dominant Short neck due to fused or cervical vertebrae Spina bifida and external canal atresia may be present
Cleidocranial dysostosis	Dominant Absent or hypoplastic clavicles Failure of fontanelles to close
Hand-hearing syndrome	Dominant Congenital flexion contractures of fingers and toes
Diastrophic dwarfism	Recessive Dwarfism Clubfoot Deformed pinnae with calcification of cartilage
Saddle nose and myopia	Dominant Severe myopia Cataracts Congenital saddle nose
Absence of tibia	Recessive Markedly shortened lower legs
Split-hand and foot	Recessive Partial syndactyly and absence of some phalanges Diminished vestibular response

Integumentary and Pigmentary Disorders

Ectodermal dysplasia, hidrotic	Dominant Small dystrophic nails Coniform teeth Elevated or borderline sweat electrolyte tests
Onychodystrophy	Recessive Short, small fingernails and toenails Strabismus Hypoactive caloric tests
Pili torti	Recessive Dry, brittle, twisted hairs
Congenital atopic dermatitis	Recessive Ichthyotic, lichenified skin in antecubital, forearm, wrist, hand, and beltline areas
Keratopachyderma, digital constrictions	Dominant Hyperkeratosis of palms, soles, elbows, and knees and ring-like constrictions of digits Constrictions of digits (constrictions begin at about age 5)
Waardenburg's syndrome	Dominant Lateral displacement of medial canthi of eyes is the only constant feature White forelock of hair Heterochromia of the irises Hypertrichosis of the eyebrows over the nasal root Hypoplasia of nasal alae
Albinism with blue irises	Dominant
Partial albinism	X-linked or recessive Progressive spotting of skin with areas of hypopigmentation and hyperpigmentation Depressed vestibular responses
Piebaldness	X-linked or recessive Blue irises Fine retinal pigmentation Depigmentation of scalp, hair, and face Strip areas of depigmentation on limbs and trunk

Table 9–1. DISORDERS THAT MAY BE ASSOCIATED WITH HEARING LOSS *(Continued)**

Lentigines	Dominant Increasing number and size of brown spots on skin Early abnormalities of genitalia Retarded growth (not always present)
Eye Disorders Myopia and mental retardation	Recessive Congenital severe myopia Mild retardation
Usher's syndrome	Recessive Progressive retinitis pigmentosa Ataxia in some
Optic atrophy and polyneuropathy	Recessive or x-linked Congenital hearing loss that progresses Progressive peripheral neuropathy Optic atrophy
Hallgren's syndrome	Recessive Retinitis pigmentosa Progressive ataxia Mental retardation (25%)
Laurence-Moon-Bardet-Biedl syndrome	Recessive Dwarfism Obesity Hypogonadism Retinitis pigmentosa Retardation
Nervous System Disorders Muscular Dystrophy	Recessive Associated retinal detachment later Progressive muscle wasting
Myoclonic epilepsy	Recessive
Opticocochleodentate degeneration	Recessive Blindness Optic atrophy Spasticity
Richards-Rundle syndrome	Recessive Congenital and severe, but also progressive, hearing loss Ataxia Muscle wasting in early childhood Nystagmus Absent deep tendon reflexes Mental retardation Failure to develop secondary sexual characteristics
Cerebral palsy	Recessive or sporadic
Cardiovascular System Disorders Jervell and Lange-Nielsen syndrome	Recessive Episodes of syncope (may cause sudden death) Prolonged Q–T interval on electrocardiogram
Endocrine and Metabolic Disorders Pendred's syndrome	Recessive Goiter, which is occasionally congenital, is usually seen in adolescence
Goiter, stippled epiphyses, and high protein-bound iodine level	Recessive Bird-like facies Pigeon breast Winged scapulae Laryngomalacia Goiter in early infancy

Table continued on following page

Table 9–1. DISORDERS THAT MAY BE ASSOCIATED WITH HEARING LOSS *(Continued)**

Iminoglycinuria	Dominant No specific physical findings
Hyperprolinemia I	Dominant Seizures Growth retardation Microscopic hematuria
Miscellaneous General Somatic Disorders Trisomy 13 and 15	Low-set pinnae Atresia of external auditory canals Cleft lip and palate Colobomas of the eyelids Micrognathia Tracheo-eosphageal fistulae Hemangiomas Congenital heart disease Mental retardation
Trisomy 18	Low-set pinnae External canal atresia Micrognathia Peculiar finger position Prominent occiput Rocker-bottom feet Cardiac anomalies Hernias Pigeon breast Low birth weight
Congenital Conductive Hearing Losses Craniofacial and Skeletal Disorders Treacher Collins syndrome	Dominant External auditory canal atresia Downward-slanting eyes with notch in lower lid Flat malar eminence Micrognathia Low-set malformed ears May have cleft palate
Otofaciocervical syndrome	Dominant Depressed nasal root Protruding narrow nose Narrow elongated face Flattened maxilla and zygoma Prominent ears Preauricular fistulae Poorly developed neck muscles
Acrocephalosyndactyly (Apert's syndrome)	Dominant High broad skull frontal prominence Exophthalmos due to shallow orbits Hypoplastic maxillae Bony syndactyly of digits
Proximal symphalangism	Dominant Stiff fingers and toes due to bony ankylosis of the proximal interphalangeal joints Stapes fixation
Otopalatodigital syndrome	Recessive Cleft palate Stubby, clubbed digits Low-set small ears Winged scapulae Malar flattening Downward obliquity of the eyes Down-turned mouth
Oral-facial-digital II (Mohr) syndrome	Recessive Nodular tongue Midline cleft lip

Table 9–1. DISORDERS THAT MAY BE ASSOCIATED WITH HEARING LOSS (*Continued*)*

Oral-facial-digital II (Mohr) syndrome (*Continued*)	Small mandible Polydactyly Syndactyly Bifid tip of nose Thick lingual frenum Widely spaced medial canthi of eyes
Oculoauriculovertebral dysplasia (Goldenhar's syndrome)	Recessive Epibulbar dermoids Preauricular appendages Fusion or absence of cervical vertebrae Colobomas of eye
Thickened ears	Dominant
Malformed low-set ears	Recessive
Preauricular appendages	Dominant Also includes preauricular pits and external auditory atresia
Madelung's deformity	Dominant Short stature, forearms, and lower extremities Posterior subluxation of ulna Limited wrist motion Exostoses of long bones and cervical ribs Funnel chest Clubfoot Spina bifida occulta Pain during periods of skeletal growth
Fanconi's syndrome	Recessive Absence or deformity of thumbs Other skeletal, heart, and kidney malformations Skin pigmentation Mental retardation Pancytopenia
Integumentary and Pigmentary Disorders Forney's syndrome	Dominant Lentigines Mitral insufficiency Skeletal malformation

Eye Disorders
  Duane's syndrome
	Recessive
	Inability to abduct eyes
	Retraction of globe
	Narrowing of palpebral fissure
	Usually unilateral
	Torticollis, cervical rib, and external ear
	  malformation may be present

Cryptophthalmos	Recessive Adherent eyelids, which hide the eyes External ear malformation

Renal Disorders
  Nephrosis, urinary tract malformations
	X-linked or recessive
	Bifid uvula
	Shortening or broadening of the distal parts of
	  fingers and toes

Renal-genital syndrome	Recessive Low-set ears Stenotic external canals may be present Vaginal atresia
Taylor's syndrome	Recessive Unilateral microtia or anotia Unilateral facial bone hypoplasia

Table continued on following page

Table 9–1. DISORDERS THAT MAY BE ASSOCIATED WITH HEARING LOSS (*Continued*)*

Syndromes in Which Congenital Sensorineural, Conductive, or Mixed Hearing Loss May Be Found

Craniofacial and Skeletal Disorders

Pierre Robin Syndrome	Dominant May be progressive Thin and elongated individual Long spidery fingers Pigeon breast Scoliosis Dolichocephaly Hammer toes
Craniofacial dysostosis (Crouzon's syndrome)	Dominant Fusion of cranial sutures Shallow orbits Prominent eyes Parrot nose Hypoplastic maxillae Relative mandibular prognathism External canal atresia may be present
Achondroplasia	Dominant Dwarfism Large head Short extremities Normal-sized trunk Saddle head Frontal and mandibular prominence Hearing loss occasionally progressive
Craniometaphyseal dysplasia (Pyle's disease)	Dominant Hearing loss also progressive Interphalangeal joints of fingers and toes Progressive whitening of nails

Ophthalmologic Disorders

Möbius's syndrome	Recessive Facial diplegia, severe but incomplete Varying degrees of ophthalmoplegia External ear malformations Micrognathia Hands, feet, or digits may be missing Tongue paralysis and mental retardation may be present

Miscellaneous Somatic Disorders

Turner's syndrome	Not inherited Low hairline Webbing of neck Widely spaced nipples Shieldlike chest Webbing of digits

Later Onset, Progressive Sensorineural Hearing Loss

Craniofacial and Skeletal Disorders

Generalized cortical hyperostosis (van Buchem's syndrome)	Recessive Onset during puberty Leonine facies Square jaw Optic atrophy
Roaf's syndrome	Not hereditary Congenital or early retinal detachment Cataracts Myopia Coxa vara Kyphoscoliosis Shortened long bones Retardation

Table 9–1. DISORDERS THAT MAY BE ASSOCIATED WITH HEARING LOSS (*Continued*)*

Ophthalmologic Disorders	
Cockayne's syndrome	Recessive Dwarfism Mental retardation Retinal atrophy Motor disturbances
Alstrom's syndrome	Recessive Onset at about age one of nystagmus and visual loss due to retinal degeneration Hearing loss beginning about age 10 Onset of diabetes mellitus in adolescence Obesity
Refsum's syndrome	Recessive Onset in second decade of visual loss and night blindness due to retinitis pigmentosa Progressive ataxia, muscle wasting, and peripheral sensory loss Ichthyosis Elevated plasma phytinic acid level
Norrie's syndrome	Recessive Congenital blindness due to pseudotumor retini Hearing loss in 25 to 30 per cent of the patients
Fehr's corneal dystrophy	Recessive Progressive visual loss to blindness by about age 40
Optic atrophy and diabetes mellitus	Recessive Progressive visual and hearing losses during first decade of life Onset of mild diabetes in first or second decade
Flynn-Aird syndrome	Dominant Progressive myopia, cataracts, retinitis pigmentosa, and hearing loss beginning in the first decade of life Ataxia, shooting pains, and joint symptoms beginning in second decade
Nervous system disorders	
Friedreich's ataxia	Recessive Childhood onset of nystagmus, ataxia, optic atrophy, hyperreflexia, and hearing loss
Myoclonic seizures	Also includes cerebellar ataxia and hearing loss
Herrmann's syndrome	Dominant Late childhood or adolescent onset of photomyoclonus and hearing loss followed by diabetes mellitus, progressive dementia, pyelonephritis, and glomerulonephritis
Severe infantile muscular dystrophy	Recessive Congenital facial weakness with resultant difficulty in eating, followed by abnormal gait, weakness of proximal and distal musculature
Sensory radicular neuropathy	Dominant Onset in late teens and early adulthood of painless ulcerations of feet and progressive sensorineural hearing loss
Acoustic neuromas	Dominant Progressive bilateral sensorineural hearing loss beginning in the second or third decade of life Ataxia, visual loss, and involvement of cranial nerves V to X may be seen Neurofibromas or café-au-lait spots are seldom seen

Table continued on following page

Table 9–1. DISORDERS THAT MAY BE ASSOCIATED WITH HEARING LOSS (*Continued*)*

Endocrine and Metabolic Disorders

Hyperprolinemia II	Dominant
	Ichthyosis
	Renal disease manifested by hematuria, calculi, renal cysts, and renal failure
Alport's syndrome	Dominant
	Onset at age 10 or later of hematuria, proteineuria, progressive renal disease, and hearing loss; worse in males than in females
	Microscopic hematuria may be detectable early in childhood
	Cataracts, spherophakia, and anterior lenticonus may be seen
Amyloidosis, nephritis, urticaria	Dominant
	Onset in teens of recurrent urticaria, with malaise and chills
	Amyloidosis precedes nephropathy and renal failure
	Progress of hearing loss parallels that of renal failure
Hyperuricemia	Dominant
	Early pubescent onset of hyperuricemia, followed by progressive sensorineural hearing loss, ataxia, and renal failure
	Cardiopathy, myopathy, and gout have been seen in some patients
Primary testicular insufficiency	X-linked or recessive or sex-limited dominant
	Early onset of blindness
	Onset by school years of "partial" hearing loss
	Normal virilization
	Small testes
	Hyperuricemia
	Elevated serum triglyceride and prebeta lipoprotein levels

Syndromes in Which Either Progressive Sensorineural or Conductive Hearing Loss Occurs

Craniofacial and Skeletal Disorders

Osteogenesis imperfecta	Recessive or dominant
	Fragile bones
	Multiple fractures with resultant deformities
	Large skull
	Triangular facies
	Blue sclerae
	Hemorrhagic tendencies (bruising and petechiae)
Osteitis deformans (Paget's disease)	Dominant
	Onset in middle age of long bone and cranial deformities and cranial nerve palsies

Table 9–1. DISORDERS THAT MAY BE ASSOCIATED WITH HEARING LOSS (*Continued*)*

Osteopetrosis (Albers-Schönberg disease)	Recessive Onset of recurrent cranial nerve palsies, especially facial, may occur in childhood Brittle but, paradoxically, sclerotic thickened bones Malignant type leads to obliteration of bone marrow, severe anemia, and rapid demise Benign type associated with large skull and mandible, excessive height, and leonine facies by teen years Occasional increased intracranial pressure
Diaphyseal dysplasia (Engelmann's syndrome)	Dominant Onset in first and second decades of life of progressive cortical thickening of diaphyseal regions of long bones and of skull Cranial nerve symptoms may be seen
Endocrine and Metabolic Disorders Hurler's (recessive) and Hunter's (x-linked) syndromes	Identical metabolic errors in which abnormal mucopolysaccharides are deposited in tissues Onset about age one in Hurler's syndrome, later in Hunter's syndrome, of coarsening of features, forehead prominence, growth and mental retardation, coarse puffy skin, and stubbiness of digits Progressive corneal opacities, hepatosplenomegaly, dementia (more severe in Hurler's syndrome), with death following within a few years
Deafness Occurring Alone Severe Congenital Sensorineural	Dominant Recessive X-linked
Moderate Congenital Sensorineural	Recessive
Congenital Unilateral	Dominant
Progressive Sensorineural	Dominant Early onset, recessive Early onset, x-linked Low frequency, dominant Midfrequency, dominant Moderate, x-linked
Progressive Conductive or Mixed Otosclerosis	Dominant Possibility of recessive inheritance in some instances has been raised

*This table was prepared by Max Bozarth, Ph.D., Consultant in Audiologic Hearing Health Care, Edina, Minnesota.

Table 9–2. OTOTOXIC MEDICATIONS CURRENTLY IN USE

Generic Name	Brand Name
Salicylates	A.P.C., Bufferin, Ascriptin, Buff-A Comp, Aspirin, Congespirin, Coricidin, Empirin, Emprazil, Equagesic, Excedrin, 4-Way Cold Tablets, Fiorinal, Midol, Monacet, Norgesic, Pabirin, Pacaps, Panalgesic, Percodan, Persistin, Robaxisal, SK-65 Compound, Supac, Synalgos, Vanquish, Zorprin.
Sodium Salicylate	Corilin, Gaysal, Pabalate
Salicylamide	Arthralgen, Bancaps, Bancaps C, Codalan, Coriforte, Dengesic, Duadacin, Duo-3x, Excedrin, Excedrin PM, Os-Cal-Gesic, Rhinex D-Lay, Sinulin
Salicylazosulfapyridine	Azulfidine, SAS-500
Salicylsalicylic Acid	Disalcid, Persistin
Streptomyces-Derived Antibiotics	
Kanamycin	Kantrex
Neomycin	Cortisporin, Myco Triacet, Mycolog, Mytrex, Neobiotic, Neodecadron, Neo-Hydeltrasol, Neo-Polycin, Neosporin, Neo-Synalar, Otocort, Otobione
Gentamicin	Garamycin, U-Gencin
Tobramycin	Nebcin
Amikacin	Amikin
Antimalarials	
Quinine	Quinidine
Chloroquine	
Chloroquine Phosphate	Aralen Phosphate
Chloroquine Hydrochloride	Aralen Hydrochloride
Hydroxychloroquine	Plaquenil Sulfate
Polymyxin-B	Aerosporin, Bro-Parin, Chloromyxin, Cortisporin, Lidosporin, Neo-Polycin, Neosporin, Ophthocort, Otobione, Otocort, Polysporin, Pyocidin-Otic, Terramycin
Colistin	Coly-Mycin
Ethacrynic Acid	Edecrin
Furosemide	Lasix
Cisplatin	
Erythromycin (in large doses)	
Minocycline	Minocin
Chloramphenicol	Chloromycetin, Ophthochlor, Ophthocort
Phenylbutazone	Azolid, Butazolidin
Sulindac	Clinoril
Ibuprofen	Motrin
Fenoprofen	Nalfon and Ampersand, Nalfon
Naproxen	Naprosyn

New Experimental Loop Diuretics that are Potentially Ototoxic

Bumetanide
Piretanide

that require outside evaluation of the patient with potential otolaryngologic problems. However, when caseload is high and time is a very precious commodity, a brief screening of hearing may be appropriate to help determine the level of specific services needed prior to referral to an otolaryngologist. Before the patient is seen by the otolaryngologist, automatic evaluation by an audiologist may be appropriate when a patient fails a screening examination and when there is an audiologist in close proximity to the otolaryngologic practice. The audiologist is concerned with helping to determine the level of hearing health care needed for the patient and has little to do with actual referral to another practitioner in the medical community.

THE GROUP OTOLARYNGOLOGY PRACTICE

The group otolaryngology practice will utilize screening to determine the level of hearing health care service that is appropriate to the patient. Screening concerns will be similar to those of the individual practitioner. With volumes of patients, the value of screenings toward practice support becomes significant and may determine the extent and depth of the screening, short of full audiologic evaluation.

THE MULTI-SPECIALTY GROUP PRACTICE

The otolaryngologist will be concerned with group public relations issues and will be active in developing good interspecialty relationships, just from a dollars and cents prospective, because such relationships build the group practice. Since each physician member building the practice has an interest in the success of his colleagues, the role of screening is enhanced. Not only does it become a mechanism for preselecting potential patients for other members of the practice but also it makes it easier for the otolaryngologist to develop a quality screening program that can serve those who have hearing problems. A variety of screening programs and a distinct protocol for each medical specialty in the group practice may be appropriate. The internist may wish to use a metabolic screening flag as a referral signal, whereas the pediatrician may wish to use a chronic middle ear effusion as a screening referral signal. Actual pure tone

screening with a portable audiometer or screening using tuning fork tests may be implemented, depending on the group practice needs and expertise available.

THE PRIMARY PRACTITIONER PRACTICE

The general practitioner, the family practitioner, the pediatrician, the gynecologist, and others in some communities serve as the primary practitioners and potential referral sources to the otolaryngologist. The primary practice person has a number of concerns relating to referrals to others. Obviously, the primary practitioner would like to treat the patient and eliminate the need for referral if possible. Some practitioners may go through rather elaborate medicine-based strategies in the treatment of some ear problems before they make a referral to the specialty service. Part of the difficulty is that these primary care people are concerned with losing their patients to the specialty physician. In setting up a screening program with a primary practitioner, it is therefore desirable for the primary practice person to understand that the otolaryngologist has a supplemental role in the patient's primary health care.

NONPHYSICIAN SETTINGS

Hearing loss is not just a concern of physicians. Indeed, long before physicians were concerned about hearing loss, educators dealing with the deaf wanted to maximize hearing so that the hearing impaired could learn and get along well in a hearing society. Educators today are concerned with hearing. School nurses may be involved in hearing screenings, but the primary motivation of public school programs is to assure that children can hear in the classroom and, if they cannot, that proper enhancement of residual hearing is obtained so that the hearing impaired can indeed learn. Educators are not opposed to an interface with physicians. They often refer to physicians for medical evaluation of hearing problems. However, as a general rule, educators are unhappy with the feedback that they receive from physicians because physicians tend to ignore the fact that it is the screening that initiated the physician consultation. To have worthwhile screening, it is necessary to provide feedback to the referral source, especially when the referral source comes from outside a medical setting. When setting up a public school screening system or modifying a system already in existence, it is expedient to build in this feedback mechanism.

There are a variety of screening agencies, besides the public schools, that have long existed for identification and referral purposes. Hearing societies, nursing home service groups, speech and hearing centers, and so on, may all have a direct interface with the otolaryngologist in some communities. If such an interface does not exist, development of screening programs to utilize the interest of such agencies can be developed. For any nonphysician groups, the feedback mechanism needs to be developed to provide the encouragement for additional, future referrals. Such feedback does not require the compromise of any patient information but rather data that show that referrals made by nonphysician agencies do take place and that hearing needs are met.

SCREENING PROCEDURES

Once a target population has been established the actual screening system used will vary depending upon that target population, the availability of nonphysician personnel time, the level of screening desired, and the equipment on hand, among other factors. The ability of the patient to give accurate information will also limit which screening procedure is utilized with which patient. A number of screening procedures are possible, ranging from relatively simple activities not requiring patient response, such as tympanometry and acoustic reflex measures, to pure tone or speech stimuli, and more complex activities requiring a high level of patient compliance. Objective measurement systems that require electroencephalogram (EEG) or auditory brainstem response (ABR) or other electrode techniques are not considered screening methods in the usual sense, since they do relate to otolaryngology entry level services. The crib-o-gram or other behavior monitoring systems of assessing hearing that require unusual equipment are also not considered screening methods for purposes of this chapter, although routine evaluation with such systems may serve as entry level mechanisms for identification of patients for otolaryngologic services. The following are simple screening systems.

QUESTIONNAIRE

There are two types of questionnaires, one completed by an observer and the other completed by the patient. For those individuals who are not trustworthy as reporters, any questionnaire is probably best answered by a family member or other individual who interacts with the person on a regular basis. This could be a parent for a young patient, a station nurse for a geriatric nursing home patient, a teacher or counselor for an institutionalized person, or a supervisor for an assembly line worker.

Specific questions asked on a questionnaire may be as simple: Does the patient have hearing problems? For a child, the questions can be tailored to some extent: Does the child hear the bathtub water running? When the child is in the other room and hears mother cooking, opening the refrigerator door, or chopping, does the child soon get under foot? Does the child turn the television up at home? Does the teacher complain that the child does not hear in the classroom? For an adult, the questions can be modified as well: In what situations does the patient find it most difficult to hear? What people are hardest to hear? When do people complain about the patient's hearing? These first questions or modifications relate to hearing acuity.

Follow-up questions relate to change in hearing function: Has the patient's hearing changed? How long has the patient noticed a difference in hearing? How long did it take for the hearing change to occur? Is it still getting worse? Does the patient's hearing change or stay the same?

It may be appropriate to inquire about balance changes at this point: Has the patient experienced dizziness or vertigo? Are the balance complaints occurring when the hearing loss occurs?

What head noises does the patient have? Is there ringing or buzzing in the ears? Is the patient having discharge from the ear? Has there been recent head trauma? What kind of work has the patient done and was there noise on the job? This last question and its answer may have to be interpreted, since people's judgment of noise exposure is not always accurate. A farmer, for instance, with years of working around farm equipment, may be exposed to substantial noise but may be oblivious to the impact of that noise on hearing. Has the patient had any major infections and been treated with medications when the hearing problems started? Has the patient been having other health problems, such as diabetes mellitus or renal disease? Is there hearing loss or other health problems in other family members (Table 9–3)?

Such a questionnaire can readily be given by nonphysician personnel. The questionnaire can be constructed to be a checklist that the patient simply marks, or it can be given verbally. If the questionnaire is routinely given by office personnel, some judgment of communication adequacy can be made as part of the questionnaire record. If any part of the questionnaire is positive for ear problems, the patient can be referred on to secondary screening (e.g., tuning fork evaluation, screening pure tones) before direct otolaryngologic evaluation.

ABBREVIATED PHYSICAL EXAMINATION

A simple look at the ear may serve as a preliminary screening. If the ear canal is obviously occluded with cerumen or foreign material or if the ear has a discharge, further evaluation is indicated. If the ear structures are atypical in shape or if atresia or other physical deviation is present, otolaryngologic evaluation is warranted. The skeletal

Table 9–3. CHECKLIST FOR DETERMINING PATIENTS WHO ARE AT HIGH RISK FOR HEARING LOSS

Directions: Circle the number of complaints that applies to the patient.

1. Problems hearing or understanding
2. Earache
3. Dizziness (like moving or falling)
4. Runny ear
5. Ringing, humming, hissing, or roaring in the ear
6. Fluctuating hearing
7. Hearing differs from one ear to the other
8. Medications result in ringing or buzzing in the ear or dizziness
9. Hearing loss in the family
10. Diabetes, kidney disease, thyroid disease in family
11. Ear stuffiness or fullness
12. Unusual sensitivity to loud sounds
13. Job history of noise exposure to machinery, assembly line, farm equipment
14. Surgical history relating to the ear
15. Others complain about the patient's hearing
16. History of ear disease
17. Wear hearing aid
18. History of head injury and changes in hearing

structure should be examined with special attention to maxillofacial structures. If these are not within the normal range, otolaryngologic assessment is indicated, particularly if features suggest an obvious hereditary syndrome. Waardenburg's syndrome, with its white forelock, dichromia of the irides, and confluent eyebrows, is a good example of a condition in which a visual screening indicates the necessity for an otolaryngologic evaluation. The patient with a cleft palate (even if repaired) also automatically warrants further evaluation if the patient is not currently being followed. Generally, this type of screening can be accomplished by nonphysician personnel.

DEVELOPMENTAL PLATEAUS FOR QUICK SCREENING BY NONPHYSICIAN PERSONNEL

In children, the failure to develop speech and language may suggest hearing loss. A number of behavioral criteria have been developed by various researchers for determining whether a child's speech and language are within the normal range. Children who fail to fall within the normal range should be evaluated for hearing loss. Otolaryngologic evaluation of the hearing loss will be needed to establish a clear etiology if possible and develop a treatment plan. Developmental plateaus have been incorporated into a number of checklists or continuum scales for quick screening purposes, such as in the Denver Developmental Screening Test, which is readily available. The Alexander Graham Bell Association's "Hearing Alert" packet is another example. This type of questionnaire may be utilized by personnel with minimal training time.

Neurologically based incoordination problems warrant otolaryngologic evaluation for verification of intact hearing function. Careful audiologic evaluation may be needed to evaluate central auditory processing problems, especially when a hearing-impaired child passes a screening test with pure tones but has definite listening problems in the home or classroom. Patients with cerebral palsy or who have suffered severe head trauma should be evaluated otolaryngologically. Again, it is the nonphysician personnel in the primary practice type of office who should be able to visually identify these kinds of problems for referral.

PURE TONE SCREENING

There are several varieties of audiometric screening procedures that can utilize pure tone stimuli. Essentially, hearing threshold levels under earphones may be obtained at several frequencies, usually in the speech range (0.5 to 3 kHz). Children who fail to hear at levels better than 25 dB HL (hearing level) and adults who fail to hear at 35 dB HL are referred for follow-up. (See Chapter 8 for a discussion of normal hearing acuity.) The referral criteria specify a hearing threshold level as the fail level. Abbreviated screening procedures may test for hearing at that level only, with patients who fail to hear at that level being directed to the otolaryngologist. Background noise levels present in any screening setting (unless the area has been satisfactorily sound conditioned) may limit the actual frequencies utilized in screening. Certainly thresholds softer than 25 dB may be difficult to obtain in many pure tone screening settings. Weber and Rinne tests at 0.5 and 2 kHz utilizing tuning forks (see Chapter 1) or the bone oscillator of an audiometer at 40 dB HL intensity may be utilized for screening purposes. In this case the background noise does not cause major problems in the interpretation of findings. Further evaluation should be performed when the Weber lateralizes or when bone conduction perception is better than air conduction perception.

SPEECH SCREENING

A speech reception threshold can be obtained under earphones if a speech circuit is present in the audiometer used in the screening process. A standard system for establishing the speech reception threshold involves finding the patient's threshold for equal-stress, two-syllable words. (See Chapter 8 for greater discussion of the speech reception threshold.) A variety of lists are available for use: the Central Institute for the Deaf (CID) W-1 series of spondees is published in a number of texts. It may be more appropriate to ask young children to identify body parts or clothing, since some children would rather point because of shyness. Some of the picture-pointing tests available for speech threshold measurement may also be desirable if time permits. For the elderly who cannot follow a repetition task, the use of responses to questions like, "How old are you?" and "Where were you born?" and "What time is it?" may be more appropriate.

The goal, as with determining pure tone threshold, is to find the softest level at which people can just function communicatively. If the screening system is not specific-threshold based, a 25-dB screen failure criterion for children and a 35-dB screen failure criterion for adults would appear adequate for speech screening. However, if the examiner is in the same room as the patient, spoken voice is too loud to really establish the hearing threshold under earphones. In such cases, speech audiometric screening is valid only when tape-recorded speech is used. When the patient is isolated from the examiner, live voice may be used for test stimuli.

SPECIAL AUDIOMETRIC PROCEDURES

There is a desire to make the screening process as objective as possible. If screening is defined as the activity that results in referral of a patient to the otolaryngologist for evaluation, many of the activities that pass for screening are automatically eliminated. Procedures that require electrodes (early, mid, or late "brainstem" responses) are automatically ruled out as screening procedures. The patients have already been preselected for evaluation, that is, the screening has already taken place; the first step in evaluation of potential hearing loss is taking place in this type of testing. Therefore, audiometric screening is seen in this chapter as a traditional audiometric or impedance/admittance status screening procedure.

TESTING ENVIRONMENT

When new programs are developed, noise problems can be explored with potential screening agencies. Testing of hearing requires a quiet area to do threshold testing. There are a number of standards that have been developed for determining adequacy of an environment for testing of hearing (Table 9–4). Certainly, formal measures of noise present in a listening environment are desirable. Generally, the settings where screening occurs should be quiet to the clinician's "normal-hearing" ear, but it is doubtful that most screening settings meet the quietness criteria set for real diagnostic hearing studies.

A quiet room for testing should be away from competing sound sources, such as windows, fans, radiators, air conditioners, ma-

Table 9–4. MAXIMUM BACKGROUND NOISE FOR HEARING TESTING USING EARPHONES*

Octave Band Center Frequencies	0.125	0.25	0.5	0.75	1	1.5	2	3	4	6	8
Band Sound Levels (dB)	34.5	23.0	21.5	22.5	29.5	29.0	34.5	39.0	42.0	41.0	45.0

*ANSI 3.1—1977 reference.

chinery rooms, and motorized chairs or tables. Rooms that have soft-textured walls or walls that are not smooth plaster are desirable. Hanging drapes or other soft materials break up the reflecting surface of the walls and do much for quieting room echoes. Fabric-covered room dividers for large rooms tend to break up many higher tone echoes. Sound absorbent ceiling tiles reduce ambient noise. If minor modifications in the room are possible, ceiling tiles that are constructed for acoustic damping may be applied to ceiling and to walls where practical. A number of companies manufacture fabric-type materials that decrease ambient noise levels relating to reverberation when they are applied to wall surfaces. However, everything from haversack material for "wallpaper" to egg cartons applied to walls and ceilings tends to make the testing environment more quiet. Simply placing carpeting on a hard tile floor does much to quiet a room, and use of carpeting on walls and ceilings can also be fruitful for noise suppression.

It is primarily high tone noise that is most suppressed by these room changes. Frequency energies below 0.5 kHz tend to be damped to a lesser degree. Thus screening at frequencies below 0.5 kHz tends to result in many false positives for referral when low-frequency "environmental" noise is present in the screening setting. Patients will not hear the test stimuli because of the masking effects of that ambient background noise. A sound survey of the testing area during a typical clinic day using a sound level meter with an octave band filter will help determine whether the testing environment is acceptable for screening. If such acoustic analysis is avoided by referral sources, which unfortunately may sometimes be the case, avoiding 0.25 kHz as a screening frequency is advised. If results of screening show that a person with otherwise normal hearing has poor hearing thresholds at 0.5 kHz, the odds are that high levels of low-band noise are present in the screening

area. Therefore, some type of educational program to upgrade the screening manager's understanding of the problem with the screening area is indicated.

IMPEDANCE SCREENING

Screening using tympanometry with acoustic reflex testing may be employed when the screening environment has high levels of background noise (see Figs. 8–23 and 8–4.) Certainly a tympanogram can be uitlized in almost any clinic without undue concern for background noise. The patient's ear status should be evaluated by appropriate medical personnel if the tympanometric pattern is not normal (i.e., there is no "peak" or the "peak" is not within $+/- 100$ ml H_2O pressure) (see Figs. 8–25 to 8–28). The otolaryngologist may seek to have primary practitioners in remote areas rescreen or monitor middle ear status for several weeks before encouraging actual otolaryngologic consultation. If the tympanogram shows no change or a worsening middle ear condition (e.g., a shifting of the "peak" toward a more negative pressure range), the referral for otolaryngologic follow-up is desirable. If the impedance audiometer comes equipped with an acoustic reflex stimulus, absence of a stapedial reflex or elevation of the reflex threshold, which is a further reason for referral, can be determined.

Screening Implementation Plan

Screening is an important aspect of hearing health care and serves as a mechanism for preselecting appropriate patients for otolaryngologic services. The model presented in Figure 9–1 follows the logic in setting up a workable screening program for an otolaryngology practice.

The first step (Box 1) is to determine what potential settings the given otolaryngology practice might relate to in terms of consults.

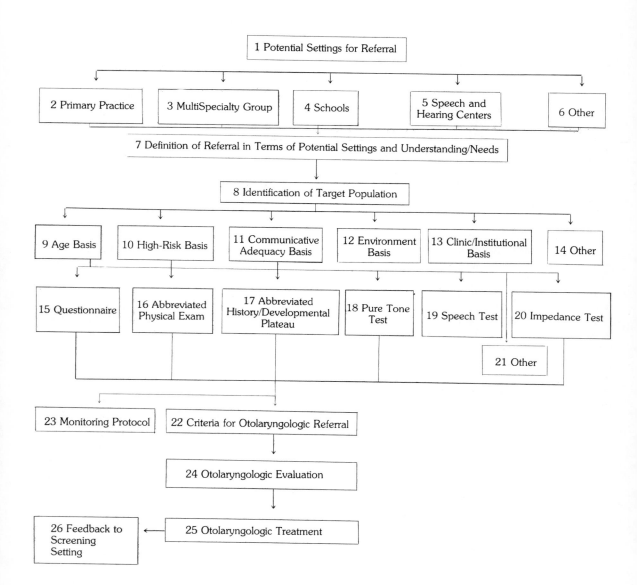

Figure 9–1. A screening model of the development of otolaryngologic referral.

Depending on the given community, a variety are possible, with many of them being feasible referral sources (Boxes 2 to 6). Once settings have been identified, marketing questions have to be addressed (Box 7), the basic question being, Why does the potential referral source want to refer to the otolaryngology practice? The question with its hypothesized answer will have to be tailored to the respective individual settings.

Contact with the potential referral source and reaching a consensus about the patient and practice benefits of referral for otolaryngologic services allows the next step in developing a screening program. Box 8 is the point at which the referral source and the otolaryngology practice jointly determine who the target population is. As discussed earlier, there are a variety of strategies for determining the target group (Boxes 9 to 14).

Once the target group or groups are determined, the variety and depth of pre-otolaryngologic screening must be determined (Boxes 15 to 21). Methods of screening chosen will reflect the settings in which the screening takes place as well as what equipment and personnel may be available for screening purposes.

The best screening program is useless without definitive criteria for referral (Box 22). Some settings may initiate a monitoring protocol (Box 23), with otolaryngologic referral occurring after failure to improve using a usual treatment strategy. When referral results (Box 24), the otolaryngologist has two equally important activities to pursue to make the screening program work. On the one hand, he must manage the medical/ surgical/rehabilitative problem of the patient, with all that that entails (Box 25), and the otolaryngologist must initiate feedback directly to the referral source (Box 26), which informs the referral source that the referral system is working and encourages referral of additional appropriate patients.

Conclusion

This chapter has reviewed some of the difficulties connected with implementation of screening programs. It has discussed the concepts of target population, setting of service, and types of procedures that are readily utilized. Finally, it has suggested a model for initiating relevant screening programs for the otolaryngology practice.

BIBLIOGRAPHY

Bradford, L. J., and Hardy, W. G. (eds.): Hearing and Hearing Impairment. New York, Grune and Stratton, 1979.

Brummett, R. E.: Drug-induced ototoxicity. Drugs 19:412–428, 1980.

Cantrell, R. W. (ed.): Noise—its effects and control. Otolaryngol Clin North Am 12:471–732, 1979.

Hopkinson, N. T., and Schramm, V. L.: Preschool otologic and audiologic screening. Otolaryngol Head Neck Surg 87:246–257, 1979.

Jaffe, B. F. (ed.): Hearing Loss in Children: A Comprehensive Text. Baltimore, University Park Press, 1977.

Northern, J. L., and Downs, M. P. (eds.): Hearing in Children. Baltimore, Williams and Wilkins Co., 1974.

Wong, D., and Shah, C. P.: Identification of impaired hearing in early childhood. Can Med Assoc J 121:529–532, 535–536, 538–542, 1979.

INDEX

Note: Page numbers in *italics* refer to illustrations; page numbers followed by (t) refer to tables.